The Antidepressant Antidote
Five Steps to Get Off Antidepressants Safely and Effectively

BETHANY BUTZER, PH.D.

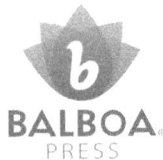

BALBOA
PRESS

Balboa Press books may be ordered through booksellers or by contacting:

Balboa Press
A Division of Hay House
1663 Liberty Drive
Bloomington, IN 47403
www.balboapresspress.com
1-(877) 407-4847

ISBN: 978-1-4525-0038-6 (sc)
ISBN: 978-1-4525-0044-7 (e)

Printed in the United States of America

Balboa Press rev. date: 11/09/2010

To David, for seeing my light when I couldn't.

Contents

Introduction

I'm sitting in the waiting room at the student health center, my eyes darting anxiously back and forth. I'm hoping with everything in me that I won't happen to see any of my friends or acquaintances. I spot a pile of old magazines and quickly grab one, pretending to look interested in how to recreate the latest fall fashions from Paris on a budget. I wish I was here for some sort of "typical" university student problem, like getting a doctor's note for a fake illness so that I can miss an exam. Instead, I'm here because my therapist thinks I might need to go on antidepressants. She couldn't prescribe the drugs herself, so I have to go see a GP. A tall, frail nurse comes around the corner and calls my name. As I walk toward her, something in me knows that I'm approaching a big decision, one that shouldn't be taken lightly.

~ ~ ~

What length would you go to rid yourself of anxiety and sadness?

I took antidepressants for 6 years.

It started when I was 20 years old. I'd recently moved away from home, and I was in a romantic relationship that was highly dysfunctional. I was also having trouble getting along with my best friend, who happened to be my roommate.

Add to this the fact that my rocky childhood was starting to catch up with me. My parents had separated when I was young, and my father eventually cut off all contact with my mother, brother, and me. My mother was an absolute sweetheart, but was extremely anxious and I seemed to have inherited her knack for worrying about almost everything. My mother remarried a man who I had a very hard time getting along with at first. My stepfather was a recovering alcoholic, was verbally abusive, and was completely blind – not in the metaphorical sense of the word, but truly blind – he had lost his sight due to a gunshot wound to the face that he suffered when someone had tried to kill him. His life circumstances gave him demons that he never fully dealt with, which caused tension between him and my family for much of his life.

Of course, things could have been worse, and I realize that my childhood wasn't as difficult as what some people have had to go through. However, I will say that my upbringing wasn't a walk in the park, and it left me with several scars that hadn't healed. So, in my early 20s, when deteriorating relationships with my boyfriend and my best friend were causing many of my issues to resurface, I decided to see a therapist.

Therapy at my university was free, and I was studying psychology, so I thought that seeing a therapist might be a good opportunity to learn about myself and get rid of some of the anxiety and sadness that I was feeling. After seeing the therapist for a few sessions, she decided to refer me to a doctor because she thought I was suffering from dysthymia and that I might need to go on medication.

I'd never heard of dysthymia before – but it sounded pretty bad! For a moment, I pictured myself being wheeled away in a Hannibal Lecter-style straightjacket. But as the therapist explained dysthymia to me, I realized that she was actually describing a relatively mild condition.

According to the American Psychiatric Association's *Diagnostic and Statistical Manual of Mental Disorders* (DSM-IV), dysthymia is a mild form of depression in which a person must have had a depressed mood on most days for at least 2 years or more, and show *two* of the following six symptoms:

- Poor appetite or overeating.
- Insomnia or hypersomnia.
- Low energy or fatigue.
- Low self-esteem.
- Poor concentration or difficulty making decisions.
- Feelings of hopelessness.

The person also cannot have suffered from a major depressive episode over the 2 year period, or a manic episode (e.g. bipolar disorder).

Looking back, I don't know if I was suffering from dysthymia or not. I was feeling down at the time, and I'm sure I mentioned to the therapist that I'd felt sad during my teenage years. My level of sadness had also never been severe. I was always able to function in my daily life, go to school, and work a steady job – and I had never been suicidal. In my opinion, however, any two of the symptoms from the bulleted list above would pretty aptly describe most second year university students!

Still, the therapist thought that I might need medication, so off to the doctor I went. The doctor spoke with me for around 15 minutes, gave me a short questionnaire that asked about my feelings of sadness, and sent me home with a trial pack of Paxil (which was one of the latest and greatest new antidepressants back in 1999).

That 20 minute appointment led to me being on antidepressants for the next 6 years.

After taking Paxil for only a few days, I had a full blown panic attack in the middle of a cafeteria on campus. I had never had a panic attack before, but I recognized the symptoms from my psychology textbooks. I went back to the doctor, who told me to cut my Paxil pills in half and get up to a maintenance dose more slowly. Many years later, I learned that increases in anxiety and agitation are quite common when people start antidepressants. My doctor never warned me about this, however, nor was I made aware of the other side effects that often come along with antidepressant use.

By the time my 6 years of antidepressant use were up, I had been prescribed three different antidepressants. First I tool Paxil, then Celexa, and finally Zoloft. I experienced a whole host of unpleasant side effects with each of these prescriptions, and I tried several times, unsuccessfully, to get off the drugs. I also never received any type of formal psychological evaluation or diagnosis. My therapist had suspected dysthymia, but her suspicions were never officially confirmed. Feeling hopeless, I resigned myself to the idea that I would need to take antidepressants for the rest of my life.

Should I have ever been put on Paxil? I don't think so. Sure, my childhood had been rocky, and I was high strung and sad sometimes. But I believe these issues could have been effectively addressed through psychotherapy and other alternatives besides medication.

Instead, I spent 6 years scouring the internet and bookstores for someone who would help me get off antidepressants. I wanted to reduce my anxiety and sadness using natural methods, and I knew I didn't want to be on antidepressants for the rest of my life. Eventually, after years of trial and error, I managed to kick my antidepressant habit for good.

The purpose of this book is to help you do the same.

The State of the Nation

According to the U.S. Centers for Disease Control and Prevention, approximately 118 million prescriptions for antidepressants are written in the U.S. every year. In fact, the number of Americans taking antidepressants rose by almost 50% between 1995 and 2002, and antidepressants are now the most commonly prescribed form of medication in the U.S., with higher prescription rates than drugs for conditions like high blood pressure, asthma, and headaches.

Approximately one in five American adults aged 18 or older have a diagnosable anxiety disorder in a given year, while 25% of Americans claim they are depressed. The World Health Organization has predicted that by 2020, depression will have a global burden that is second only to heart disease. And while antidepressants are necessary in some cases, many doctors, psychiatrists, and psychologists agree that these drugs are being overprescribed for a variety of conditions, such as fatigue, sleep difficulties, PMS, and mild sadness or stress.

Primary care doctors are extremely busy, and don't often have the time or experience necessary to give patients a full psychological evaluation. Instead, many patients are sent home with a pack of pills, when psychotherapy could be equally or even more effective than antidepressants. Add to these statistics the fact that multi-billion dollar pharmaceutical companies are advertizing the marvelous effects of the newest type of antidepressants – the Selective Serotonin Reuptake Inhibitors (SSRIs) like Prozac – and you have a recipe for disaster that has led to millions of people being prescribed antidepressants unnecessarily.

There are more prescription drugs available now than ever before. These drugs are supposed to cure every possible problem, from erectile dysfunction to shyness. We are bombarded by TV and magazine ads displaying beautiful, happy people skipping through fields of joy because they have taken their magic pill that has fixed everything. Well, everything except for the anal discharge and heart palpitations that are occurring as a result of the magic pill, but they don't show that part on TV.

Pharmaceutical companies have even skewed research to make it look like antidepressants are more effective than they really are. These companies have also promoted the idea that antidepressants correct a chemical imbalance in your brain, despite the fact that this hypothesis has never been scientifically proven. In fact, some countries outside the U.S. have banned pharmaceutical companies from promoting this misleading idea.

As Joseph Glenmullen, M.D., points out in his book "The Antidepressant Solution," people who are anxious or depressed are fed all sorts of information that hasn't been confidently proven by modern science. For example, these people are often told that they have a genetic condition, despite the fact that studies attesting to the genetic basis of psychological disorders have not stood the test of time.

People are also often told that their anxiety or depression is a "disease." In fact, no psychological condition meets the strict medical criteria necessary to be called a disease. To call a condition a disease, the cause of the condition or an understanding of its physiology must be known. Many people are also led to believe that anxiety and depression are life-long diseases that necessitate an indefinite use of antidepressants. However, this is a relatively new belief that only started being widely disseminated when SSRIs broke onto the scene in the 1990s. Before that, only the most severe forms of depression were thought to be a life-long problem.

Please know that I'm not an embittered conspiracy theorist who is making this up. The shady behavior of pharmaceutical companies when it comes to antidepressants has been well documented both legally and in the press. For a detailed account of these issues, I suggest the books *"Prozac Backlash"* and *"The Antidepressant Solution"* by Joseph Glenmullen, M.D., as well as *"The Antidepressant Era"* by Dr. David Healy.

To make matters worse, antidepressants can cause a host of side effects – things like low sex drive, dry mouth, and night sweats. Antidepressants have even been linked to more serious side effects such as disfiguring facial tics and an increased risk of suicide (see Joseph Glenmullen's book *"Prozac Backlash"* for a detailed description of these side effects).

I would be happy to hazard a guess that many of the people who are currently taking antidepressants probably don't want to be on them. A simple Google search reveals hundreds of websites and chat rooms filled with people seeking the answer to one question:

"How can I get off antidepressants?"

Eleven years ago, I was asking this same question.

Why Did I Write This Book?

I wrote this book because I've heard stories like mine over and over. There are so many people who go to a doctor for some sort of mild condition, and leave with an antidepressant. As I mentioned earlier, antidepressants are sometimes necessary in severe cases, but these drugs are often prescribed to people who don't really need them – people who could resolve many of their issues through other approaches. Joseph Glenmullen, M.D., author of the book *"Prozac Backlash,"* believes that 75% of the people who are currently taking antidepressants could significantly reduce their dose or stop taking antidepressants completely (with the help of their doctor) by using alternative approaches to manage their depression and anxiety, such as psychotherapy and lifestyle changes.

I agree with Dr. Glenmullen that many safe and effective alternatives exist to treat depression and anxiety. There are also a multitude of clinical studies attesting to the effectiveness of these alternatives. Of course, you will need to consult with your doctor to decide whether or not you're ready to begin reducing your antidepressant dose. But I will tell you right now that I believe there is a high likelihood that you can eventually live an antidepressant-free life. It might not happen right away, and it will take some hard work and commitment on your part, but it can be done.

I have now been off antidepressants for 5 years, and I know that I will never need to take them again for the rest of my life. How can I be so sure? Because I know that whenever I feel anxious or sad, I can always draw on the tools outlined in this book.

My genuine hope is that this book will help you on your personal journey toward a calm, happy, and purposeful life. I realize that words like "happy" and "purposeful" might seem like airy fairy feelings that are completely out of reach – but I promise that if you are truly committed to helping yourself feel better, you *will* experience happiness, purpose, and a whole lot more.

A Few Disclaimers

Before I go any further, however, there are a few things that I need to make clear. First, as I've mentioned several times, I am *not* completely against the use of antidepressants. I think that in some cases, antidepressants are absolutely necessary to help people get on their feet and function in society. There are also many pharmaceutical drugs that help people immensely with problems like schizophrenia and bipolar disorder.

I will say, however, that I believe many people today are being given medication when they don't need it, as a quick fix. This isn't necessarily the fault of doctors, as they are understandably busy and need to get patients in and out of their offices as quickly as possible. In some cases, patients themselves are also looking for a quick fix, because they don't want to put in the time and effort necessary to go to psychotherapy or change their lifestyle.

Despite my opinions on the over-prescription of antidepressants and the big bad pharmaceutical companies, I am not your doctor or therapist and I believe that these people should be involved in your journey to get off antidepressants as much as possible, as they can provide you with additional support when you need it. Before reducing your antidepressant dose, *please* consult with your doctor to make sure that you're ready.

I'm also not a medical doctor, so I can't provide advice about the exact milligram dosage reductions that you should make. And I'm not a neuroscientist, so I've refrained from providing detailed descriptions about precisely how antidepressants work in your brain. For information on recommended dosage reductions, as well as the biological aspects of antidepressants, please see the book *"The Antidepressant Solution"* by Joseph Glenmullen, M.D.

If at any time while you're trying to get off antidepressants you feel even the slightest urge to hurt yourself or others, contact someone for help and get back on antidepressants if necessary. As you will see, it took me several tries before I finally managed to kick my antidepressant habit. You can always try again at a point when you're feeling more stable. It's much better to take your time when trying to go off these drugs than to end up ruining your life, or someone else's life, because you weren't ready to begin lowering your dose.

I also need to make it clear that when I use the term "antidepressant" in this book, I'm referring to today's most popular antidepressants, which are the Selective Serotonin Reuptake Inhibitors (SSRIs) and the Serotonin and Noradrenalin Reuptake Inhibitors (SNRIs) mentioned previously. Currently, these antidepressants include Paxil, Zoloft, Prozac, Celexa, Lexapro, Luvox, Effexor, Pristiq, Cymbalta, and Serzone. Note that many of these antidepressants have generic or medical names that might be different from the names listed here. Ask your doctor to identify exactly what type of antidepressant you're taking.

Older classes of antidepressants, such as monoamine oxidase inhibitors (MAOIs) and tricyclic antidepressants, are not the focus of this book. For recommendations on how to taper off these older types of antidepressants, please see the book *"The Antidepressant Solution"* by Joseph Glenmullen, M.D.

This book is also written with an adult audience in mind, and thus doesn't apply to reducing antidepressant doses in children or adolescents. The effects of antidepressants in children and adolescents are still not well understood, which is why I need to limit the scope of this book to an adult population. For those who are interested, *"The Antidepressant Solution"* by Joseph Glenmullen, M.D., provides suggested SSRI and SNRI tapering programs for children and adolescents.

Please also keep in mind that the five steps outlined in this book are not necessarily meant to be followed from step 1 to 5 in chronological order. Some people might start by getting help, then kick their antidepressant habit, then move on to letting go and choosing wisely. Others might make life-changing choices first while they're still on antidepressants, then start tapering their dose. Feel free to follow these steps in whatever order feels right for you. I will suggest, however, that you start with step 1, which involves enlisting the help of professionals and friends, before you go off antidepressants.

Finally, I need to highlight that this story represents my personal journey toward antidepressant freedom. Parts of it might resonate with you, while other parts may not. I know that during my journey, I felt horribly alone. No one in my social circle had been on antidepressants for years and was trying to get off them. Throughout this book, I share snippets of my story so that you won't feel alone in your journey. Take what you will from my story and use it in a way that's helpful for you.

My ultimate purpose in writing this book is to help you feel supported as you try to get off antidepressants, and to empower you with resources to help you choose the approaches that work best for you. If I could sit down with each and every person who's struggling with antidepressant use, trust me, I would. But alas, the best I can do is share my experiences and hope that my words will support you.

You can do this – I know you can. There were times when I felt like I would have to be on antidepressants for the rest of my life. But I managed to get off the drugs and so can you. I stand by and support you on your journey, and your journey starts here.

Many health and wellness books quote philosophers and poets like Plato or Rumi. While I appreciate all the masters who came before me, I can't help but quote a more contemporary source. As the band Rage Against the Machine so aptly put it in their song *"Guerilla Radio:"*

"It has to start somewhere, it has to start sometime. What better place than here, what better time than now?"

Start your journey toward antidepressant freedom. I'm here by your side, and we'll get through it together.

List of Resources

At the end of each chapter in this book, I list any resources that were mentioned in the chapter so that you can find all of the information in one place.

- *"Prozac Backlash"* by Joseph Glenmullen, M.D.
- *"The Antidepressant Solution"* by Joseph Glenmullen, M.D.
- *"The Antidepressant Era"* by Dr. David Healy.

Chapter 1
Step 1 – Get Help

I open my eyes and it's dark. The room is spinning. *I'm sweating, and I think I'm going to throw up. I swing my legs over the side of my bed and I take a deep breath – why do I feel so weird? I hadn't been drinking any alcohol, and I went to bed nice and early. Then the revelation comes creeping through the fog of my sleepy thoughts: it's the antidepressants. I'd just started taking the pills from my trial pack of Paxil. I'd taken a pill before bed, and now I was feeling more anxious than I'd ever felt before being on the medication. A surge of nausea catches itself in the back of my throat and I panic. I'm living with 11 other people in a student housing unit, and none of them know that I've started taking antidepressants. I have nowhere to turn, no one to talk to, it's the middle of the night, and I feel horribly alone.*

~ ~ ~

I'm not going to beat around the bush: getting off antidepressants was one of the most challenging things I've ever done. I've been through my fair share of trials and tribulations, and I've achieved some pretty significant milestones in my life. But the process of getting off antidepressants ranks up there as one of the most difficult things that I've ever had to go through.

As you'll see in Chapter 2, reducing your antidepressant dose can bring with it a host of physical and psychological side effects. This is why I *strongly* recommend that you seek both personal and professional help before, during, and after you try to get off antidepressants. This help can come in several forms – through a romantic partner, through friends, through your doctor, through therapy, and even through alternative medical approaches like naturopathy.

The bottom line is this: don't go through this alone. I know it can be hard to admit to people that you're taking antidepressants. Throughout the entire 6 years that I was on antidepressants I felt ashamed, embarrassed, and terrified that the people who were close to me might find out that there was something wrong with me and that I didn't really have it all together. It took me 5 years just to build up the courage to write this book! My reluctance to share my truth with others is one of the main reasons I tried several times, unsuccessfully, to get off the drugs, and why I ended up on antidepressants for so long.

I hate to sound cliché, but it really is true that no person is an island. I liken it to when members of Alcoholics Anonymous (AA) enlist the help of a sponsor. When you're going off antidepressants, you need someone you can call in the middle of the night when you wake up sweating and scared. You will need the support of your closest friends, family, and professionals to get through this.

Your Romantic Partner, Friends, and Family

I'm sitting on the couch with my new boyfriend. We've spent a wonderful Saturday together and we're about to watch a movie. He grabs his bowl of popcorn and flashes me his winning smile, dimples and all – a smile that I subsequently came to adore.

"I know we've only known each other for a few weeks," he says, "but I just want to say how lucky I feel. You're smart, you're good looking, and you're funny. It's almost like you're too good to be true."

I turn my head and stare out the window so that he can't see the pained expression on my face. Little did he know that I'd been on antidepressants for 4 years, and I was planning on making my third attempt to go off them in the next few weeks. In my mind, I'd convinced myself that there was something seriously wrong with me. Why couldn't I manage to get off these drugs? He was right – I was too good to be true.

I turned to face him and was caught off guard again by his smile – so genuine and full of hope for our new relationship. In that moment, something in me shifted. Maybe the glass of wine that I'd had was going to my head, or maybe, just maybe, I'd finally decided to trust someone with what I was going through.

"Well, I'm definitely not perfect," I said as I played with a thread that had come loose on the couch. And then it all came spilling out. I told him the story of how I ended up on antidepressants, and I mentioned that I was planning on trying to go off them.

He listened intently, and as I was talking I envisioned the reaction that I expected from him. He would go running for the hills and never look back. I mean really, we were in our 20s, in the prime of our lives, and I appeared to have the emotional baggage of a 40 year old man going through a midlife crisis.

When I finished talking, he paused for a moment – a moment in which I figured he was scaling my apartment to find the fastest escape route. Instead, he put his hand on mine and said very matter of factly:

"Ok, we'll do this together. When do we start?"

~   ~   ~

When I first went on antidepressants, I kept it a secret from everyone. On the surface, I looked like I had it all together. I'd graduated top of my class in high school, I was valedictorian, and I received a hefty scholarship to start me off in university. Throughout my undergraduate education, I was again top of my class, winning almost every scholarship and award that I could. I'd started to make a name for myself in the psychology department, and on the outside my life appeared fantastic. The professors at my university thought highly of me, I was reasonably attractive, I had a boyfriend, I had an active social life, and I had a family that cared about me.

Beneath the surface, however, I was anxious, sad, and felt alone. I was preoccupied with getting good grades and making everyone proud of me. The inklings of my not-so-ideal childhood haunted me, and I had very little confidence or self-esteem. Despite the fact that I had several close friends, I didn't feel that I had anyone who I could confide in about being on antidepressants. I was ashamed and embarrassed that I needed a drug to make me happy.

So I kept my antidepressant use to myself.

Aside from my boyfriend at the time, not a single one of my friends or family members knew that I took a little pink pill every day to stay sane.

A few days after I had a Paxil-induced panic attack in the cafeteria at my university (described in the Introduction) I was scheduled to write a big exam. I was terrified that I would have another panic attack in the middle of the exam, so I made an emergency appointment at the student health center. I explained to the doctor what had happened to me, and he gave me a note that would allow me to defer the exam and write it at a later date if needed. Instead of sharing my fears with my friends or family, I went to the exam the next day with the doctor's note tucked safely in the front pocket of my backpack. I never used it. On the surface, I looked like a typical student writing an ordinary exam. But inside I was screaming.

Later, when I decided to try to go off antidepressants for the first, second, and third time, I continued to keep everything that I was going through a secret. I would run into the washroom when I started to experience withdrawal effects, and try to "wait it out," hoping that no one had noticed that I was acting strange. I would pray while I was driving that the tingling sensations in my head and hands wouldn't cause me to get in an accident.

And each of the times that I tried to go off antidepressants without telling anyone, I ended up right back on them.

Despite my training in psychology, I truly underestimated the importance of social support when dealing with life's difficulties. I was aware of studies showing that the support of friends and family is a huge buffer against stress, but I was so paralyzed with the fear of people finding out that I wasn't perfect that I decided to attempt one of the hardest things I would ever do in an isolated bubble.

Little by little over the 6 years that I was on antidepressants, I started telling the odd person about it. Sometimes this happened by accident, like when my mom found out. I was about to get my wisdom teeth pulled, and my mom was sitting in the dentist's office with me. The dentist walked in with my chart, and very nonchalantly asked "So are you on any other medication besides Celexa?" Little did he know that his apparently innocuous question exploded like a bomb in my mom's unsuspecting ears.

I'm not going to lie – when my mom later asked me what Celexa was and I admitted to her that I'd been taking antidepressants for years, it wasn't like I suddenly felt a million times better. It was hard to admit to my mom that I'd been in therapy and been prescribed a psychiatric drug. She was worried, like all moms would be, and the last thing I wanted to do was worry her. There were also some people who weren't overly accepting of my antidepressant use when I told them about it. For example at one point when I tried to explain to a new boyfriend that I was acting strangely because I was trying to get off antidepressants, he told me that he "didn't want to hear any more sob stories" that would excuse my behavior.

However one thing I was expecting to happen when I started telling people that I was on antidepressants didn't happen: the apocalypse.

In my mind, the second I admitted to my mom or anyone else that I was on antidepressants, the world as I knew it would end, possibly due to a large catastrophic event. Perhaps I had a grandiose view of my self-importance, but

I was absolutely convinced that the world would end if I admitted to anyone that I was taking SSRIs or that I was attempting to get off them.

But guess what? My world didn't end, and yours won't either. Over time, I started admitting to more and more people that I was taking antidepressants. I didn't suddenly broadcast it to every available ear, but I did share it with close friends and romantic partners when the moment seemed right.

The amazing thing that I noticed as I started to share what I was going through was that many of my friends were facing similar demons. Their situations weren't identical to mine, but my friends and family had their own issues to deal with. They had panic attacks, eating disorders, felt sexually inadequate, were afraid to come out of the closet, had serious problems with their romantic partners, and several other difficulties that kept them up at night. And by and large, they were going through these issues alone. They felt isolated, like no one truly understood what they were going through.

The "new boyfriend" that I described at the beginning of this section eventually became my husband. He didn't run for the door when I admitted that I was on antidepressants, and he was willing to support me in my effort to get off them. It wasn't a walk in the park for him as he tried to help me through my emotional ups and downs, but his support was an extremely important factor in my ability to finally kick my antidepressant habit. He helped me realize that it was ok to feel sad and anxious sometimes, and that this didn't make me insane. He also helped me see that I didn't need medication to keep me mentally stable.

Perhaps I was lucky in the sense that I had a very supportive romantic partner and equally supportive friends. You might think there's no one out there who would support you in your journey toward antidepressant freedom. However I truly believe that there is always someone out there who is willing to support us. Even if you have absolutely zero friends (which I suspect is highly unlikely if you're honest with yourself), the advent of the internet has brought alternative avenues for support. Join an online chat group of people who are trying to get off antidepressants. Even a "virtual friend" can act as a rock of support when you need it.

Your Doctor

I eyed my doctor anxiously, wondering how she was going to react to my big revelation. I'd been on antidepressants for over 2 years, and I was going to try to go off them. I wanted her help, but I didn't quite know how to ask for it. I started out by asking her how long most people have to take antidepressants for. She smiled and said, "In my experience many people end up taking antidepressants for a very long time, and some have to be on them for the rest of their lives. It's kind of like a diabetic taking insulin. The insulin helps the diabetic with their problem, so why stop taking it? If you have a chemical imbalance in your brain and the antidepressants are helping to regulate that, then often it doesn't make sense to stop taking the medication."

This wasn't the answer I'd been hoping for. But maybe I was like a diabetic who needed insulin – my brain was messed up and I needed drugs to make me "normal." Maybe I would just have to resign myself to being on antidepressants for the rest of my life. In the end, I said nothing about my desire to get off antidepressants. I mentioned that I was having some annoying side effects, like night sweats, dry mouth, and low sex drive, and I left with a prescription for a new type of antidepressant – Celexa – that supposedly had fewer side effects.

~   ~   ~

It might be understandable that I was scared to tell my friends and family about my antidepressant use and my desire to get off the drugs. The strange part is that I was even afraid to tell my own doctor that I wanted to get off antidepressants! This led to several failed attempts to get off the drugs, where I would try to quit cold turkey and mistake my withdrawal symptoms for the original symptoms that had led to me being on the medication in the first place.

I think the main reason I was scared to tell my doctor that I wanted to go off antidepressants was that I was afraid of her response. I feared that she would try to talk me out of it and feed me another story about antidepressants being to depressed people what insulin is to diabetics. This wasn't necessarily my doctor's fault. She was a GP and she didn't have a lot of training in how and when to prescribe psychiatric drugs.

When I changed universities to attend graduate school, I started seeing a new doctor. This doctor became one of my closest allies in my quest toward antidepressant freedom. He was busy, and he didn't have a ton of time to spend with me, but instead of just refilling my prescription every time I went to see him, he took the time to ask me questions. Questions about how I was feeling, how long I had been taking antidepressants, and if my side effects were starting to get on my nerves. In this environment, I felt free to contemplate the wild and crazy idea that maybe I could live a happy life without antidepressants. When I eventually admitted to him that I was considering going off the drugs, he gave me suggestions for how to taper off slowly to ensure that I would experience as few withdrawal effects as possible.

I urge you to *please* work with your doctor as you try to get off antidepressants. Don't decide to stop taking your medication cold turkey simply because your prescription runs out. I'm not a medical doctor and I can't tell you exactly how to begin reducing your dose, but for recommended tapering schedules for today's popular antidepressants, see the book "*The Antidepressant Solution*" by Joseph Glenmullen, M.D. I also recommend sharing Dr. Glenmullen's book with your doctor.

In the end, I eventually came to see antidepressants as less like insulin and more like a band aid – a temporary fix for an underlying problem that wasn't going to go away until I ripped the band aid off and allowed the wound to breathe.

The Role of Therapy

I'm 7 years old and I'm walking home from school. My grey dress is making my legs itchy and I can't wait to take it off when I get home. I wonder what's for dinner and contemplate whether I should play with my cabbage patch dolls or My Little Pony. I open the front door and make my way to the kitchen. My mom is sitting on a chair by the kitchen table and my aunt is standing beside her. I realize that something's wrong and my little heart starts to race at a rabbit's pace.

I walk toward my mom and put my hands on her knee. "Mommy what's wrong?" I ask.

She's crying so hard that words don't come out of her mouth. My aunt kneels down beside me and puts her hands on my shoulders, turning me to face her. "Your dad isn't coming home" is all I remember her saying.

After this, my memory comes in brief flashes. I'm watching TV as my aunt checks to see if I'm ok...then a wave of recognition hits me as I realize that daddy really isn't coming home – ever. Then a surge of anxiety comes over me as I wonder how my mom, brother and I are going to live without him.

At first we saw dad on the odd weekend. Then he made his presence known only through Christmas and birthday cards. By the time I was 10 years old, he cut off all contact with us, even though he only lived 15 minutes away.

The last time I saw him, he was sitting on his motorcycle at a red light. I was with my mom, shopping for shoes for my grade eight graduation. My mom turned and whispered to me "That's your dad." My eyes followed the low growl of the idling Harley. I saw the familiar brown work boots and leather vest that he always wore. My memory of his face had faded, and I was eager to see what he looked like. As my eyes moved up, I realized he was wearing a helmet with a tinted visor. The only image I saw as he slowly looked away from me was my own – the pained face of a little girl trying to catch a glimpse of the father who had left her behind.

~   ~   ~

I believe that a lot of the time we end up on antidepressants because we want a quick fix for our problems. We want a band aid that's going to cover everything up and make it go away. It makes sense that we crave this quick fix, because often the pain that we're experiencing is intense. The reality of the situation, however, is that your problems are *never* going to go away until you take active steps to deal with them. And one sure fire way to end up on antidepressants for life is to avoid dealing with the issues that got you in this situation to begin with.

I ended up in therapy in the first place because I was having issues. Now whether or not those issues were serious enough to warrant a prescription for antidepressants is a whole other matter, but suffice it to say that therapy played an important role in helping me sort out my problems. As I mentioned before, I hadn't had an ideal childhood by any stretch of the imagination, and a troubled childhood often serves as a catalyst for the types of issues that cause people to go on antidepressants.

I must say that the process of being a therapeutic client came somewhat naturally to me. I really liked talking about and analyzing my problems, and I learned a lot about myself in the years that I spent in therapy. By the age of 26, I had pretty much tried every therapeutic approach I could find. I had talked to an empty chair that was supposed to represent my childhood self. I had talked about my issues while holding two egg-shaped pods that vibrated in alternating rhythms in my left and right hands. I had studied my Jungian shadow self. I had taken self-esteem and anti-stress workshops. And I had filled out countless thought records as homework for my cognitive behavioral therapy.

The only problem was this: when my antidepressants were working well, I didn't feel the need for therapy anymore.

So I ended up in a cycle where I would go to therapy, start opening my wounds, feel overwhelmed, go on antidepressants, and then stop going to therapy. Then I would go through a few months when I was on antidepressants but not in therapy, and I would be feeling great, so I would try to go off the antidepressants. Then I would end up feeling overwhelmed again and back in therapy, then back on antidepressants, and the cycle would continue.

Please hear me when I tell you that antidepressants are *not* a substitute for therapy. They are a band aid that's covering up what's really going on for you. There is almost *always* a reason for our symptoms of anxiety and depression – whether we're aware of the reason or not. Anxiety and depression are often symptoms of an underlying problem, in the same way that a fever is often a symptom of an infection. Taking antidepressants to mask your symptoms is like taking Tylenol for a fever – it makes you more comfortable but it also means that you never get to the root of the problem. This leaves you vulnerable to relapses in the future. Joseph Glenmullen, M.D., describes this point perfectly in his book *"Prozac Backlash:"*

"In no other brand of medicine would we tolerate treating symptoms without investigating and treating the underlying problem. Can one imagine patients with pneumonia being put on aspirin indefinitely and not receiving any other treatment? Why should we tolerate this kind of 'treatment' for psychiatric conditions?"

Think about what led you to go on antidepressants in the first place. Were you feeling anxious? Depressed? Irritable? What was it that made you feel that way? Did you experience a significant life stressor or something else that triggered your feelings? Sometimes these underlying issues might not be clear to you, or you might simply think that you don't have any problems. Therapy can illuminate what's going on for you, and help you move beyond it.

In the end, you need to speak to someone about the reason(s) you ended up on antidepressants in the first place before you try to go off them. Just because the antidepressants make you feel better, this doesn't mean your issues have been magically resolved. Sure, friends and family can act as a support network as you try to get off antidepressants, but there's something different about talking to a completely unbiased, neutral observer. Your therapist can help you examine the reasons why you (or your doctor) felt that you needed to be on antidepressants in the first place, and help you move forward.

Numerous studies have found psychotherapy to be as effective (or even *more* effective) than taking antidepressants, particularly for mild to moderate depression and anxiety. Some studies have even replicated this result for *severe* depression and anxiety. When it comes to the long-term effectiveness of psychotherapy versus antidepressants, several studies have shown that people who go through psychotherapy are less likely to have a relapse of their depression or anxiety than people who only take antidepressants. Psychotherapy helps you develop a resistance to future bouts of depression and anxiety because it arms you with the mental awareness and tools to keep your symptoms at bay. Antidepressants, on the other hand, simply mask your issues, which means these problems can easily return in the future when you go off the drugs.

People tend to give five main excuses for avoiding therapy. Let me address each of these excuses in turn:

- **You don't like the therapist**. Not every therapist is going to be a perfect fit for everyone. There are multiple different types of therapists and therapies out there, which are described in more detail below. If you don't like your therapist, keep trying until you find someone who is a good fit for you.
- **Therapy makes you uncomfortable**. In many ways, this is the point of therapy. Avoiding the issues and feelings that make you

uncomfortable is a sure fire way to end up on antidepressants for good. Decades of studies have shown that we often need to process and work through our issues in order to overcome them. Popping a pill every day to sweep your issues under the rug is not the answer.

- **The therapy isn't going anywhere**. I will admit that at times when I was in therapy, I felt like I was talking in circles. I seemed to bring up the same issues over and over, without coming to any resolution. But again, this is all part of the process of working through your problems instead of brushing them to the side. Sometimes you need to repeat yourself over and over to notice your dysfunctional patterns. Looking back over the many years that I spent in therapy, I can now see the bigger picture. Each session was a tiny step that got me to where I am today. At the time, I might have felt like I was going in circles, but I was actually discovering who I really was.

- **You can't afford it**. Many insurance programs cover psychotherapy. If you don't have insurance, or if your insurance runs out, almost every town or city has clinics that offer psychotherapy on a sliding scale basis, or even for free. A simple Google search or perusal of the Yellow Pages can help you find these clinics.

You don't need to talk to someone who has been on Oprah for the therapy to be effective.

- **You don't have time.** I find this argument against therapy one of the hardest to deal with. I firmly believe that you *always* have enough time for your well-being. If you don't feel like you have the time right now, take a few things off your plate and *make* the time. You owe it to yourself. What do you have in life without your health and well-being? We'll talk more about making smart choices in Chapter 4, but for now, I urge you to make yourself a priority.

What's the bottom line here? Find a therapist who you connect with, and continue to see this person even if the therapy brings up uncomfortable feelings or issues.

I've sat in countless therapists' waiting rooms feeling embarrassed to be there. Making the decision to see a therapist can be difficult. But you need to get over any fear or embarrassment and just do it. You would be amazed at how many people are secretly getting therapy and not telling anyone about it. It's much more common than you think. And while it might be hard to talk about your problems, I guarantee that it will get you closer to living an antidepressant-free life. Also, make sure you continue to see your therapist even after you get off antidepressants. This can help you become resilient against future stressors, and keep you from having to go back on the drugs at a later date.

Talking to a therapist might not be as easy as popping a pill every day, but the results are well worth it.

Types of Therapists

When it comes to the question of what type of therapist to seek out, the choices can be overwhelming. There are entire books written on this topic alone, but I give a brief description of several types of therapists below. The services provided by these professionals are often covered by health benefit and insurance packages (usually up to a certain dollar amount per year). This is another great reason to seek out therapy. If it's already covered by your insurance or health care plan, what do you really have to lose?

- **Clinical or Counseling Psychologists.** These professionals typically have a Ph.D., Psy.D. or Ed.D. In most provinces and states, psychologists can't prescribe medication, so they tend to focus on various forms of psychotherapy, and will refer clients to medical doctors or psychiatrists if they feel medication is required.
- **Psychiatrists** typically have an M.D., and are able to prescribe medication. Psychiatrists receive very similar training as regular medical doctors; however they also complete specialized

internships to learn about psychological disorders.

- **Psychopharmacologists** are a subset of psychiatrists who have an M.D., but who only prescribe medication and do not practice psychotherapy.
- **Social Workers.** These professionals usually have an M.S.W. (Master of Social Work) degree. Social workers provide therapy to a variety of populations such as families and people with addictions. Social workers also often help former inpatients integrate back into the community.
- **Psychiatric Nurses** are typically registered nurses who can have a B.Sc., B.A., or M.A., and who specialize in helping psychiatric patients during inpatient care.
- **Counselors.** This is a broad term that encompasses people with a variety of types of education and training. Counselors can have an M.A. or M.Sc. degree, or a specific degree in counseling from a college or university. Counselors often work with issues around everyday adjustment, such as marital or career problems. However some counselors also work with more severe populations.
- **Life Coaches.** Life coaching is a relatively new approach that involves working with clients to achieve their goals. In contrast to traditional

therapy, which often focuses on circumstances in the past that have led to current issues, coaching tends to be future-focused, with the coach and client working together to achieve outcomes that the client desires. Several life coaching certification programs exist, however most life coaching services are not covered by health care or insurance packages.

Types of Therapies

Another area that can overwhelm people when they're trying to find a therapist is the multitude of different therapeutic approaches that exist. Again, there are entire books written on this topic alone, but I've briefly outlined a few different types of therapy below.

- **Psychodynamic Approaches.** Popularized by Freud in the early part of the 20th century, psychodynamic approaches aim to help clients uncover the unconscious aspects of their psyche that are causing their psychological and physical problems. Psychodynamic approaches use methods like free association, where the client talks about everything that comes into their mind. Many forms and variations upon psychodynamic approaches exist, such as ego analysis and time-limited dynamic psychotherapy.

- **Humanistic-Experiential Approaches.** These forms of therapy focus on the client's subjective experience, paying particular attention to the client's current emotions and irrational thoughts. This type of therapy focuses less on unconscious motivations or past issues, and more on the client's free will to make responsible choices in the present. Types of humanistic-experiential therapy include client-centered therapy, existential therapy, and Gestalt therapy.
- **Cognitive Behavioral Approaches**. These approaches hinge on the idea that our thoughts and feelings influence our behaviors. Cognitive Behavioral Therapy (CBT) focuses on addressing and changing a client's irrational thoughts and feelings, which will subsequently change their behaviors. CBT is particularly effective at treating both anxiety and depression. For more information on CBT, as well as helpful exercises to reduce your anxiety and depression, see the books *"Mind Over Mood: Change How You Feel By Changing the Way You Think"* by Dennis Greenberger, Ph.D. and Christine Padesky, Ph.D., and *"Beat the Blues Before They Beat You: How to Overcome Depression"* by Robert L. Leahy, Ph.D.

- **Eclectic and Integrative Approaches**. It's relatively rare to find therapists who subscribe to only one type of therapy. Many therapists draw on several approaches, depending on a client's particular situation. In fact, separating the types of therapy as I've done above creates a somewhat arbitrary distinction, but can be helpful for those who are trying to understand the various theoretical approaches to therapy.

This brief description does not do justice to the vast amount of information out there on different types of therapy. If you're interested in learning more, ask potential therapists what type of therapy they offer so that you can make a well-informed choice.

What Type of Therapist and Therapeutic Approach are Best for You?

You might try several different therapists and therapeutic approaches – I know I did. If a particular counselor or form of therapy doesn't work for you, keep trying new therapists and approaches until you find something that clicks. Trust me when I say that your search will be well worth it in the end.

No single therapist provided everything that I needed, but over several years of seeing different therapists, I slowly started to unravel the knots that had been tied in my psyche, and gradually came to a point where I could survive without antidepressants or therapy. But before you get to that point, you have to start somewhere. Start with one therapist and see how it goes. If it doesn't work out, try someone else.

Above all else, don't stop going to therapy just because the antidepressants have lulled you into a false sense of security. Keep at it with therapy and over time you will put together the puzzle pieces that make up who you are. For a directory of therapists in the U.S. and Canada, visit www.therapists.psychologytoday.com. You can also visit www.crhspp.ca/findlist.php for a directory of Canadian psychologists.

Alternative Medicine

One important lesson that I learned in my journey toward antidepressant freedom is that the physical body and the mind are intimately connected. When getting off antidepressants, it's important to work on more than just your mental well-being – taking care of the physical body is important too.

Throughout my journey, I tried several herbal remedies that I had heard were helpful for anxiety and depression, like St. John's Wort and Valerian. I was tired of being on a synthetic drug and I was hoping that I could switch my antidepressant with something a little more "natural." I soon realized that this simple switcheroo was not going to work. Many herbal remedies state that they should not be taken at the same time as antidepressants, but I couldn't seem to stay off the antidepressants long enough for the herbal remedies to take effect.

Feeling frustrated, I decided to make an appointment with a naturopath. I was hoping he or she could help me taper off antidepressants and find a more "natural" remedy for my anxiety and sadness. I opened the yellow pages and called the first naturopath who had a reasonable looking ad.

That one frustrated phone call led to a series of events that helped me get off antidepressants for good.

My naturopath referred me to a style of yoga that was extremely effective at reducing my anxiety. As you'll see in Chapter 3, yoga provided a natural way for me to calm my anxiety and reduce my feelings of sadness and insecurity. But for now, I want to focus on several alternative medical approaches that contributed to my antidepressant freedom.

Naturopathy

Naturopathic medicine has become increasingly popular in recent years. This form of medicine combines scientific knowledge with natural approaches to help diagnose, treat, and prevent illnesses. Naturopathic doctors go through rigorous training programs that include 3 to 4 years of pre-medical training, followed by a 4 year program at an accredited naturopathic college.

After they graduate, naturopaths have to pass a 3-day licensing exam as well as provincial- or state-regulated oral and written exams.

The main goal of naturopathic medicine is to help patients reach a state of well-being that encompasses the physical, emotional, and spiritual components of their life. In essence, a naturopath helps your body heal itself, which then prevents future illness down the road. Many insurance programs cover the cost of naturopathic consultations. Some insurance plans even cover the cost of any supplements (herbs, vitamins, etc.) that the naturopath prescribes to you, although this type of coverage is less common.

The main difference I noticed between visiting a naturopath versus my regular family doctor was my naturopath's focus on my well-being from a holistic perspective. She not only prescribed supplements for my physical and mental well-being, but she also suggested lifestyle changes and other things to help me out. Typically, your first visit with a naturopath is an hour long, at which point they ask you all sorts of questions about your background, lifestyle, and current symptoms. Subsequent visits are typically a half hour long, which gives the naturopath plenty of time to check in on how you're doing.

When you're going off antidepressants, I suggest that you work with your regular doctor (or whoever prescribed the antidepressants) and a naturopath at the same time.

Your doctor can help you gradually reduce your dose, while your naturopath addresses the broader physical and mental issues that you may have. I found this combination of traditional western medicine and naturopathy to be highly effective in helping me get off antidepressants.

Several studies have attested to the beneficial effects of supplements like St. John's Wort, Omega Fatty Acids (i.e. Fish Oil), Valerian, Kava, and other naturopathic remedies for depression and anxiety. Recent advances in orthomolecular medicine, which involves bringing the body into balance using natural substances like vitamins and minerals (see www.orthomed.org), has also shown promise in reducing the symptoms of depression, anxiety, and even schizophrenia. I saw my naturopath regularly for around 3 years, during which time she prescribed numerous different supplements to me, and I still see my naturopath whenever my body gets out of balance or I get ill.

I'm not a naturopath, so it's beyond the scope of my qualifications to suggest which types of naturopathic remedies and herbs might work for you. Everyone is different, so I suggest that you book an appointment with a naturopath to find out for yourself. It's important, however, to make sure that you don't just swap a herb or a supplement for your antidepressant to make you feel better. Naturopathic doctors use herbs and supplements as *temporary* solutions to help your body heal itself and to make you less prone to illness (both mental and physical) in the future.

It's also important to keep in mind that although a supplement might be described as "natural," this doesn't mean it's not powerful. This is why I always recommend that people see a naturopath instead of just going to a health food store to pick up some herbs. Naturopathic remedies can strongly affect your system, which is why it's crucial to consult with a naturopath before taking herbs or supplements. In fact, some of the supplements that are available in health food stores for depression, like St. John's Wort, can interact negatively with SSRIs – making it essential to consult with a naturopath *before* taking these types of remedies.

Of course, some people believe that naturopaths are "witch doctors" who prescribe ineffective supplements to their patients. As I mentioned above, many studies are emerging that attest to the beneficial effects of naturopathy. However I will admit that in the beginning, having been trained as a research scientist, I found myself skeptical of whether or not naturopathy could really work for me. I only represent a sample of one person, but I can say without a doubt that naturopathy played a crucial role in helping me get off antidepressants.

You might be thinking that my positive response to naturopathy simply represented a placebo effect. In other words, I believed that the supplements would work, so they worked. But you know what? Even if all the benefits that I received from naturopathy were placebo effects (which I doubt), in the end these effects helped me get off antidepressants, which is really all that mattered. I would take a placebo effect any day if it meant that I could spend the rest of my life antidepressant-free. Plus, much of the cost of seeing a naturopath was covered by my insurance program, so I really had nothing to lose.

I strongly suggest that you book an appointment with a naturopath. If it doesn't end up working for you, then so be it. But you owe it to yourself to try as many options as possible if you really want to get off antidepressants. To learn more about naturopathic medicine and to find a naturopath near you, go to www.naturopathic.org.

Ayurveda

Many naturopathic doctors use Ayurveda in their practice, but I wanted to highlight Ayurveda separately because I found it extremely beneficial in helping me get off antidepressants. Ayurveda is an ancient medical system that was developed in India approximately 5000 years ago. "*Ayur*" and "*veda*" are two Sanskrit words that mean "knowledge of living." Ayurveda is often referred to as the "sister science" of yoga, and it's believed by many to be the basis of several therapeutic approaches like aromatherapy, massage, energy therapy, and yoga postures.

Ayurveda defines health as complete physical, mental, emotional, social, and spiritual well-being. The Ayurvedic system was originally proposed by ancient sages, but is currently being confirmed by quantum physicists and molecular biologists. So while Ayurvedic concepts may seem "airy fairy" to some of you, I strongly suggest that you keep an open mind, because this ancient system of medicine works.

The Ayurvedic system holds that humans are intimately connected to the rest of the natural world. For example, many of the base elements that exist in a tree or an ocean also exist in the human body. The physical body is thus seen as an extension of our environment, meaning that we affect and are affected by everything around us. This connection is believed to exist on a deep energetic level – we are not solid beings that are separate from our environment. Instead, we are a pattern of energetic vibrations that exist in a sea of natural intelligence. Although ancient, this view is being confirmed by quantum physicists, who have recently shown that matter is more aptly described as waves of energy than discrete particles.

According to Ayurveda, the natural intelligence that governs the world around us also governs our bodies, from our cells to our digestive and nervous systems. We experience disease when this natural flow of energy is blocked. Ayurveda helps us heal ourselves by bringing the body back to its natural intelligence when it gets out of balance. In essence, Ayurveda focuses on the uniqueness of each individual and aims to get at the underlying cause of symptoms instead of focusing only on the symptoms themselves.

The Ayurvedic system proposes that the five elements (air, fire, water, earth, and ether/space) combine into three life-forces that are present in everything that exists in the natural world, including minerals, plants, and animals/ humans. These three life-forces, called "*doshas*," support all of our bodily functions, and bring about disease in the body when they are out of balance. The three doshas include:

- *Vata*. This is the air dosha, which governs our senses, mental balance, nervous system, and movement. It controls the flow of energy in our bodies and helps us adjust to change.
- *Pitta*. This is the fire dosha, which is responsible for all chemical and metabolic transformations in the body. It helps us digest our food, and also helps us process our intellectual and emotional experiences.
- *Kapha*. This is the earth dosha, which holds all aspects of our physical structure together (e.g. cells, tissues, organs, etc.). Kapha also regulates the energy of our thinking and emotions, and governs our immune system.

Each human being is believed to possess all three doshas in varying amounts. For example, some people have one dosha that's predominant. Others might have two doshas that are predominant, or have relatively equal amounts of all three doshas. If you would like to determine your doshic constitution, you can fill out a questionnaire at www.ayurveda.com/online_resource/constitution.pdf.

In a broad sense, Ayurvedic principles hold that when any of our doshas are out of balance, we experience disease. In order to cure and prevent disease, we need to engage in practices that help us bring our doshas back into balance.

To bring these principles to life, I'll use myself as an example. I tend to be vata-dominant, with moderate pitta and low kapha. In other words, I'm small-boned, I get cold easily, I have dry skin, and I have an active, restless mind (this is just a small example of what typically makes up a vata-dominant constitution). When life throws me a curveball, I tend to get anxious, stressed out, and I develop digestive problems. When I first saw my naturopath, my vata dosha was out of balance, and I needed to bring more pitta and kapha into my constitution. Pitta, the fire dosha, helps with things like digestion, while kapha, the earth dosha, helps you feel calm and grounded.

As another example, my husband tends to be kapha-dominant. He's very laid back, has a medium build, tends to have oily skin, and is always warm. When his kapha gets out of balance due to life stressors, he tends to put on weight, get lethargic, and develops respiratory problems like sinus infections. In these situations, he needs to bring more vata and pitta into his constitution to give him energy and stamina.

The principles of Ayurveda suggest practices that can help bring your doshas into balance when they get out of whack. For example, when I have too much vata in my system, I need to eat warm, easy-to-digest foods, and engage in grounding practices like gentle yoga and meditation. When the weather gets cold in the fall, it's especially important for me to stay warm by bundling up and wearing fluffy slippers around my house (which is mostly hardwood). When my husband has too much kapha, he needs to get moving through things like exercise, and he needs to eat light, cold foods like raw fruits and vegetables.

These examples only highlight the tip of the iceberg when it comes to Ayurvedic practices. The moral of the story is that by paying attention to the balance of the doshas in your body, you can do practical things to help reduce your anxiety and depression.

I highly recommend dealing with a naturopath who is familiar with Ayurveda when you're getting off antidepressants. In their book *"Healing Depression the Mind-Body Way: Creating Happiness with Meditation, Yoga, and Ayurveda"* Nancy Liebler, Ph.D. and Sandra Moss, M.S.P.H. outline three depression archetypes based on the doshas: airy depression, burning depression, and earthy depression. These authors go on to suggest specific practices that are best suited to each type of depression. I highly recommend their book to those of you who are interested in exploring Ayurvedic principles further.

Ayurveda is an immense field of study, with entire books devoted to it. Obviously I can't cover everything about Ayurveda here. If you're interested in learning more, speak with your naturopath, or go to www.ayurveda. com.

Reiki and Thai Massage

Two final forms of alternative medicine that I found particularly helpful when I was getting off antidepressants were Reiki and Thai massage. Reiki is a Japanese form of energy work. The word "*Rei*" means "God's wisdom or the Higher Power" and "*Ki*" means "life force energy." During a Reiki session, the practitioner puts their hands on (or just above) your body, and allows healing energy to pass through them into your body. A Reiki session is typically an hour long, although you can receive longer or shorter sessions as well.

Now before you close this book because you think I've gone off the deep end, I encourage you to keep reading. Reiki is not a religion or some sort of cult – it's a very safe, peaceful, and calming way to experience healing. As I mentioned in the section on Ayurveda, even quantum physicists are beginning to show that our world is fundamentally made up of energy. Reiki practitioners tap into this universal energy and channel it into the areas of your body that need healing. Reiki helps "unclog" energy blockages that can throw your doshas out of balance, thereby leading to healing.

Reiki is growing in popularity, and was even featured recently on the Dr. Oz show. Dr. Oz's wife is a Reiki Master, and he expressed his belief that the principles of Reiki hold the foundation for the next evolution of the Western medical model. Personally, I've found Reiki to be extremely calming and healing, and I believe this form of energy work greatly helped me get off antidepressants.

Now the skeptics among you might feel that the beneficial effects of Reiki represent a placebo. This is possible, and I leave it up to you to decide whether or not Reiki works for you. It has definitely worked for me, and I suggest that you try it before you dismiss it. For more information, feel free to visit www.reiki.org.

I also found Thai massage to be quite helpful in my journey toward antidepressant freedom. Thai massage is similar to typical massage therapy, except the practitioner moves your body into gentle stretching positions while they do the massage, which helps rebalance energy blockages in the body. Thai massage practitioners also often teach their clients relaxing breathing techniques to enhance the healing effects of the massage. The client lays down the entire time (on their back, stomach, and/or side), while the practitioner gently moves the client's arms and legs into various positions depending on their needs. To learn more, visit www.thaimassage.com.

A Few Final Words on Getting Help

In this chapter I've described many forms of help that you can use as you go off antidepressants, from doctors to naturopaths to energy work. I highly recommend sampling from these approaches, figuring out which ones work for you, and using them throughout your journey. No single practitioner or modality has all the answers to everything. And while it can take a fair bit of time to visit several different practitioners on a regular basis, the results are well worth it.

The alternative to seeking help is to continue taking an antidepressant every day. This is a quick and easy fix, but is also very likely to leave you depressed or anxious again when you try to get off the medication. Actively seeking help for your issues can be uncomfortable, time consuming, and can cost money – which is why I always say that the journey to get off antidepressants is not for the faint of heart. It takes hard work, courage, and determination to face your demons and devote financial resources to your well-being. But in the end this is the only way for you to develop resilience against anxiety and depression, and to live an antidepressant-free life.

List of Resources

- *"Prozac Backlash"* by Joseph Glenmullen, M.D.
- *"The Antidepressant Solution"* by Joseph Glenmullen, M.D.
- *"Mind Over Mood: Change How You Feel By Changing the Way You Think"* by Dennis Greenberger, Ph.D. and Christine Padesky, Ph.D.
- *"Beat the Blues Before They Beat You: How to Overcome Depression"* by Robert L. Leahy, Ph.D.
- Directory of therapists in the U.S. and Canada: www.therapists.psychologytoday.com.
- Directory of Canadian psychologists: www.crhspp.ca/findlist.php.
- Orthomolecular Medicine: www.orthomed.org.
- Naturopathy: www.naturopathic.org.
- Ayurveda: www.ayurveda.com.
- *Healing Depression the Mind-Body Way: Creating Happiness with Meditation, Yoga, and Ayurveda"* by Nancy Liebler, Ph.D. and Sandra Moss, M.S.P.H.
- Ayurvedic Constitution Questionnaire: www.ayurveda.com/online_resource/constitution.pdf.
- Reiki: www.reiki.org.
- Thai Massage: www.thaimassage.com.

Chapter 2
Step 2 – Kick the Habit

*I*t's the middle of the night and my back is on fire. I feel heavy, and I can't seem to drag myself away from the flames. The heat wraps itself around my torso and moves up toward my face. I'm asleep, but not dreaming. There's only darkness and burning. I pull my heavy arms out from under my blanket to try to cool down. As my movement rouses me slightly, I realize that I'm sopping wet, and the heat that had enveloped me dissipates into a clammy cold. Feeling more awake and somewhat curious, I move my hands back under the blanket to feel my stomach. For what seems like the hundredth night in a row, I'm absolutely soaking wet. Night sweats and hot flashes are supposed to happen to pre-menopausal women in their fifties.

But I'm only 22 years old.

My sheets are drenched, and the hair at the nape of my neck is starting to wrap itself into curls from the condensation. *These night sweats had become an all too common occurrence in my life. Needless to say, things could get embarrassing when a boyfriend happened to sleep over. How was I supposed to explain the fact that at least three times per week I woke up in the middle of the night covered in sweat, to the point that I had to change my pajamas? I would try to very quietly slip out of bed without my boyfriend noticing, while I blindly searched for a new set of pajamas. In the morning, I would wake up feeling highly unsexy in my hastily chosen pair of flannels from the 90s.*

But what other choice did I have? I was on antidepressants and I didn't want to admit it to anyone – not even my own mother, let alone my romantic partners. The antidepressants gave me night sweats, along with a host of other side effects, but I could put up with the side effects because the pills made me happy, right?

~   ~   ~

Before I get into the topic of actually kicking your antidepressant habit, I should explain a bit about how antidepressants work. As I've mentioned before, I'm not a medical doctor or a neuroscientist, so my description here is relatively simple and brief. Those who are interested in getting more information on the biological aspects of SSRIs should refer to the book *"Prozac Backlash"* by Joseph Glenmullen, M.D.

SSRIs work by blocking the re-uptake of serotonin by neurons, which are the cells in your brain. Neurons have microscopic gaps in between them called synapses. Your brain cells communicate with each other by releasing chemicals called neurotransmitters, such as serotonin, into these synapses.

As an example, one neuron will release serotonin into the gap between itself and another neuron. Receptors on the second neuron absorb some of the serotonin, which completes the signal. The original neuron then "cleans up" any serotonin that's left in the synapse – a process that's called re-uptake. SSRIs work by blocking this re-uptake process. By blocking re-uptake, SSRIs cause an increased amount of serotonin to linger between your brain cells, which results in prolonged serotonin signals in your brain.

When people first go on an SSRI, they sometimes experience side effects as their brain adjusts to these increased levels of serotonin. These side effects often diminish as the body adapts to the increased serotonin, however some people continue to experience side effects for the entire time they take SSRIs.

Going Off SSRIs

So what happens when a person tries to go off SSRIs? This is where the story gets interesting. Pharmaceutical companies suggest that a very small percentage of people (around 10-20% according to some pharmaceutical advocates) experience something they call "discontinuation syndrome." This "discontinuation syndrome" involves unpleasant side effects that result from lowering one's SSRI dose. In reality, however, the number of individuals experiencing this "discontinuation syndrome" is not that small.

As an example, a pair of studies done at the Massachusetts General Hospital and Harvard Medical School found that Effexor, Paxil, Zoloft, and Prozac caused withdrawal effects in 78%, 66%, 60%, and 14% of patients, respectively. Notice that I used the term "withdrawal effects" in the previous sentence, not "discontinuation syndrome." I changed my wording here because the symptoms associated with "discontinuation syndrome" are more accurately and truthfully described as withdrawal effects. In fact, by coining the term "discontinuation syndrome," pharmaceutical companies have purposely avoided using the word "withdrawal" because of its association with addiction.

Chat rooms and message boards on the internet are filled with posts by people who have tried to go off SSRIs, but experienced a host of withdrawal symptoms. In his book "*The Antidepressant Solution*," Joseph Glenmullen, M.D. describes 28 psychiatric and 58 physical withdrawal symptoms that can occur when people reduce their SSRI dose. These withdrawal symptoms have been published in numerous case reports and large scale studies of SSRI withdrawal reactions.

Psychiatric SSRI withdrawal symptoms can include things like crying spells, irritability, low energy, and anxiety, just to name a few. Physical SSRI withdrawal effects can include symptoms like nausea, dizziness, electric zap-like sensations in the brain or body, and headaches. Notice that many of the psychiatric SSRI withdrawal symptoms resemble conditions that people are often prescribed antidepressants for in the first place, such as anxiety and depression. Often, these side effects are misinterpreted as being the original symptoms that caused the individual to go on SSRIs in the first place. Many people become so frustrated with these withdrawal effects that they end up back on antidepressants unnecessarily.

Personally, I experienced several uncomfortable withdrawal effects when I went off SSRIs. I was lightheaded, nauseous, and I felt tingling sensations in my hands and up the back of my neck. These sensations then caused me to feel anxious, which made me think that I needed to be back on the pills. Like many others, I became trapped in a cycle of trying to get off SSRIs, only to find myself back on them because I couldn't handle the withdrawal effects.

Are SSRIs Addictive?

I wholeheartedly believe that SSRIs are physically and psychologically addictive, and there are many doctors and therapists out there who agree with me. Pharmaceutical companies, on the other hand, play with semantics by calling antidepressant withdrawal "discontinuation syndrome." My personal experiences, and the experiences of thousands of others like me, suggest that we are dealing with much more than a slight "discontinuation syndrome" that's experienced by a rare percentage of the population. As Joseph Glenmullen, M.D. describes in his book "*The Antidepressant Solution:*"

> *"Withdrawal is the process of stopping or tapering off antidepressants and the characteristic symptoms that can occur as a result. Not all patients who develop withdrawal symptoms become addicted, or dependent. Addiction occurs when patients suffer such intolerable or incapacitating withdrawal symptoms that they are forced to restart the drugs, put the dose back up, or taper off them more slowly. Patients are then dependent on the antidepressants for as long as it takes to wean off the drugs."*

In other words, antidepressants become addictive when a patient has such a hard time getting off the drugs that they need to go back on the medication, increase their dose, or taper off more slowly. According to this definition, I was definitely addicted to antidepressants.

For those who don't believe that antidepressants are addictive, I pose this experiment: after you've finished reading this chapter, re-read the stories that describe my experiences, and replace the words "antidepressant" and "SSRI" with the word heroin, cigarettes, or alcohol. In reading this revised version of my story, you would probably conclude that I had a pretty severe substance abuse problem. When I tried to go off antidepressants, I craved them, both physically and psychologically. I felt like I needed just one more pill to make all my nasty feelings go away. And I had to wean off antidepressants in the same way that many addicts wean off their drug of choice.

As Dr. Glenmullen describes above, not everyone becomes addicted to antidepressants. However, there are many people out there who have felt addicted to SSRIs. In his book "*The Antidepressant Solution*," Dr. Glenmullen describes a two-part BBC expose that reported on the addictive characteristics of Paxil in 2002 and 2003. After these programs aired, their help lines received over 65,000 calls from viewers who wanted more information. In addition, over 1,300 viewers sent emails in response to the show, and the BBC website received more than

120,000 hits. Obviously, more than just a few people are interested in the withdrawal effects that can occur when reducing their antidepressant dose.

Tips to Kick Your Antidepressant Habit

I'm at a party, trying to fit in and have fun. No one knows that I've been on antidepressants for the past 3 years, and that for the past week I've been slowly trying to wean myself off them. I figure a night out will do me some good and get my mind off the pills. I smile and I laugh with my friends, while just below the surface I'm aching to tell someone how I really feel. I keep getting random tingling feelings in my hands – like electric shocks jolting through my fingers. And then, just when I think I'm finally letting go and having a good time, I feel a cold, tingling sensation creeping up the back of my neck that sends electric currents into my head. I start to get anxious. Can people tell that I'm feeling weird? Am I acting strange? What if I pass out in the middle of the party?

I go to the bathroom to collect myself. I sit on the side of the bathtub with my head between my hands and think to myself "If only I was still on antidepressants. Then I wouldn't have to feel this way. I would feel happy and normal and not like I was going to pass out every five minutes. I think when I get home I'm going to start taking my full dose again. That's the only answer. I just can't live like this. I want my life back."

~   ~   ~

I've lost count of how many times I experienced some variation of the story above when I tried to get off antidepressants. After awhile I started to believe that I was never going to be able to kick my antidepressant habit. I was going to be an antidepressant "lifer" and there was nothing I could do about it.

I'm writing this book because I was wrong.

My doctors, who told me that I might need to be on antidepressants for the rest of my life, were also wrong. Sure, some people probably do need to be on antidepressants for a long time, especially those with severe depression who could inflict harm on themselves or others if they were to stop taking their medication. However, it isn't necessarily the case that *you* will need to be on antidepressants for the rest of *your* life, even if a well-intentioned doctor told you so.

I don't blame my doctors for what happened to me. My doctors had the best intentions and were trying to prepare me for the fact that I might have to take mood altering drugs for the rest of my life. My doctors were extremely busy and had a million other patients to see that day, and I couldn't expect them to sit with me for an hour to truly evaluate my situation.

I believe that if you suffer from mild to moderate depression or anxiety, you probably don't need antidepressants to reduce your symptoms, and you definitely don't need to be on the drugs for the rest of your life. As I mentioned previously, Joseph Glenmullen, M.D., author of *"Prozac Backlash"* believes that 75% of the people who are currently taking antidepressants can significantly reduce their dose or stop taking antidepressants completely (with the help of their doctor and other lifestyle changes).

As I mention throughout this book, there are several safe and effective alternatives to taking antidepressants. For now, let's focus on how you can make the transition to antidepressant freedom as painless as possible.

Make Sure You're Ready

Keep in mind that right now might not be the best time for you to get off antidepressants. In his book *"The Antidepressant Solution,"* Joseph Glenmullen, M.D. suggests five key criteria to establish whether a patient is ready to get off antidepressants.

The patient must meet *both* criteria 1 and 2:
1. Their original condition has improved substantially.
2. They are in a relatively stable, calm period in their life.

In addition, preferably the patient meets one or both of criteria 3 and 4:

3. They have grown psychologically in ways that make them less vulnerable to the condition that the drug was made to treat.

4. Their life circumstances have changed so significantly that the original circumstances that made them depressed/anxious are no longer present.

In addition, meeting criteria 5 and 6 adds further weight to the decision:

5. They have significant side effects that contribute to their desire to go off the medication, or necessitate going off.

6. They want to go off the antidepressant rather than stay on it indefinitely because of concerns about long-term side effects and risks, especially if they no longer need the drug.

If you're currently going through a major life stressor, or you haven't done any psychotherapy to uncover why you ended up on antidepressants in the first place, now might not be the best time for you to go off antidepressants. Instead, work on improving and stabilizing your life circumstances by using the help outlined in Chapter 1 before you try to taper off antidepressants.

Of course, the list above is not exhaustive, and it's extremely important to consult with your doctor before you begin reducing your dose. Together, you and your doctor can decide whether or not you're ready to go off antidepressants.

Don't Quit Cold Turkey

If you don't take any other piece of advice in this entire book, please at least follow this small nugget of wisdom: do not quit antidepressants cold turkey. Weaning off SSRIs slowly is *extremely* important, because quitting cold turkey can cause withdrawal effects to be much worse.

The reason that weaning off antidepressants slowly is important is because most SSRIs have a relatively short half-life. A drug's half-life refers to the length of time it takes for half of the drug to wash out of your body after you stop taking it. In other words, if an antidepressant's half-life is 48 hours, then 48 hours after your last dose, half of the drug has washed out of your body. The short half-life of most SSRIs means that they clear out of your body fairly quickly. When this happens, your brain and body must rapidly adjust to the quick drop in the drug, which is what causes withdrawal symptoms.

As Joseph Glenmullen, M.D., describes in his book "*The Antidepressant Solution*," Effexor has a very short half-life – only 5 hours – which is why people can experience quite severe withdrawal reactions within hours of missing their full dose. Cymbalta, Pristiq, Luvox, Serzone, Paxil, Zoloft, Lexapro, and Celexa also have relatively short half-lives of between 11 and 35 hours. Prozac has the longest half-life of all the SSRIs at 4 to 6 days, which is why Prozac is associated with the fewest withdrawal symptoms.

Most people who experience withdrawal effects when going off SSRIs tend to notice these symptoms within 2 to 5 days after reducing their dose – *even if they don't stop their dose completely.* In other words, even reducing your Paxil dose from 40mg to 20mg per day can potentially cause withdrawal effects. These symptoms usually go away within 2 to 3 weeks, but can return when the person makes subsequent dosage reductions. People's responses to reducing their SSRI dose vary widely. Some people don't experience any withdrawal effects, while others experience extreme, debilitating withdrawal symptoms. This is why it's *extremely* important to work with your doctor while you taper off antidepressants slowly.

In his book *"The Antidepressant Solution,"* Joseph Glenmullen, M.D., suggests making dosage reductions every 3 to 5 weeks to give your brain cells time to adjust to the decreased levels of the drug. For people who experience extreme withdrawal effects, it can sometimes take months to completely wean off antidepressants. However it's very important to be patient with yourself at this stage. It's better to take awhile to get off the drugs than to rush and end up back on them.

Each person is different, so it's important to consult with your doctor to determine an appropriate antidepressant tapering program for you. In his book, *"The Antidepressant Solution,"* Dr. Glenmullen provides recommended tapering programs for many of today's popular antidepressants. I strongly recommend that you buy Dr. Glenmullen's book, and show it to your doctor. In his book, Dr. Glenmullen also provides a helpful checklist for monitoring your withdrawal symptoms, which can be downloaded at www.drglenmullen.com/AS Appendix 1.pdf. Using this checklist to monitor your withdrawal symptoms can help your doctor identify whether your symptoms are in fact withdrawal effects, or whether they represent a return of your original depression or anxiety. As Dr. Glenmullen points out in his book, there are a few key features that tend to distinguish SSRI withdrawal effects from the return of your original depression or anxiety:

- **Timing.** Psychiatric withdrawal effects, such as crying spells and increased anxiety, tend to appear quickly – within a few days of stopping your medication or reducing your dose. A depressive episode, on the other hand, usually takes one month or more to manifest.

- **The co-occurrence of physical withdrawal symptoms.** If a person is experiencing physical withdrawal symptoms, such as dizziness and nausea, at the same time as the psychiatric symptoms appear, then this strengthens the case that the psychiatric symptoms represent a withdrawal effect.

- **Time course of symptoms**. SSRI withdrawal symptoms usually peak within 7 to 10 days after a dosage reduction and clear up within 2 to 3 weeks. If you can tolerate mild to moderate withdrawal symptoms, it's usually worth it to see if your symptoms will eventually fade. A psychiatric condition, on the other hand, typically doesn't go away after 2 to 3 weeks.
- **Disappearance of symptoms when the SSRI is reintroduced**. When a person's withdrawal reaction is so severe that they have to put their dose back up, the withdrawal symptoms usually begin to dissipate within hours, and are often completely gone within 24 hours. If a person is unsure about whether their psychiatric symptoms represent withdrawal, they can take a "test dose" of their SSRI to see if their symptoms fade. When a person experiences a relapse of their actual psychiatric condition, SSRIs usually take 2 to 4 weeks to take effect. If, after taking a test dose, the person's symptoms begin to fade quickly, then this increases one's confidence that the symptoms represented withdrawal.

The bottom line is this: don't stop taking antidepressants cold turkey simply because your prescription runs out or because you don't feel like taking them anymore. I tried that, and my withdrawal symptoms were awful. To get off antidepressants successfully, I started by slowly tapering my dose, in consultation with my doctor. I did this by cutting my pills in half for awhile (you can get cheap pill cutters at most drug stores), then cutting them into quarters. Talk to your doctor about a weaning regimen that would work best for you based on your dose.

If You Can, Keep Pushing Through.

Despite the fact that I weaned off antidepressants slowly, I still experienced withdrawal effects. My withdrawal effects were probably not as bad as they would have been if I'd quit cold turkey, but they were still a struggle to deal with. In the end, I had to put up with the side effects and keep moving forward, all the while reassuring myself that soon they would go away. In the same way that the shakes and irritability of nicotine withdrawal dissipate over time, so too did my antidepressant withdrawal symptoms.

It wasn't easy to put up with the withdrawal effects. There was always a little voice inside my head that pressured, "Just go back to your regular dose and you'll feel better. All these nasty feelings will go away and then everything will be ok." It was so hard not to listen to that voice. And I will admit, many times I did listen and I went back up to my regular dose.

The reason I titled this section "*if you can*, keep pushing through," is that I don't want you to think you're some kind of a failure if you can't handle the withdrawal effects and you end up back on your full dose. The fact of the matter is that right now just might not be the best time for you to get off antidepressants. You can always go back up to your full dose and try again later. I tried several times to get off antidepressants, and I was finally able to do it when all the stars aligned properly for me with regards to my dose, my doctor, and the various forms of help that I was pursuing.

If your withdrawal symptoms are so severe that you can't function in your daily life, or you get the urge to harm yourself or others, please see your doctor immediately and get back on the medication. If, on the other hand, your withdrawal symptoms are mild enough that you can bear them for a few days or weeks, then it's worth trying to tolerate them to get off the medication once and for all.

In the end, I finally managed to push through the withdrawal effects and come out on the other side. Now when I say that I "came out on the other side," I don't want you to picture me rising like a phoenix from the ashes into a beautiful heavenly place, because it wasn't like that at all. Sure, the withdrawal effects were finally gone. But in their place was something scary that I hadn't experienced in a long time: feelings.

Allow Yourself to Feel

I wake up one morning after weaning off antidepressants and for the first time in a long time I don't feel dizzy and I'm not covered in sweat. A flutter of excitement passes through me as I realize that the withdrawal effects are starting to pass. It's Friday, and my new boyfriend is coming from out of town to take me to the movies. The day goes by quickly and I feel fantastic – I've finally beat the antidepressant demon that had its claws in my back for years.

We go see a romantic comedy – the type of movie that only a new boyfriend is willing to put up with to make a good impression. I find myself laughing at the movie, really laughing, for the first time in awhile. But then comes the classic point in all romantic comedies before the quirky hero comes to save the eccentric heroine. For a brief moment, the audience feels that all is lost, and a contemporary (but not too cheesy) love song starts to play.

I swallow, and then I swallow again – hard. "What's this choking feeling creeping up the back of my throat," I wonder to myself. "Is it another withdrawal effect? I thought I was done with those!"

The love song hits its climax, the heroine looks out her window into the dark winter night, and I feel a strange burning sensation in the corners of my eyes. "Oh God, this is so embarrassing," I say to myself. "What's going on with me?"

And then it happens: I start to cry. Big fat tears rolling down my face – even as the hero comes running down the wintry street with a bouquet of wilting flowers. Then it hits me: I can't remember the last time I cried.

~   ~   ~

After my withdrawal effects dissipated, I started to experience a whole host of feelings that I hadn't felt in a long time. Don't get me wrong – I didn't feel completely numb while I was on antidepressants (although some people do). I laughed sometimes, and I cried sometimes, but it was as if the feelings didn't come from a very deep place while I was on the medication. When I went off the drugs, there were times when I felt completely assaulted by my feelings. They felt so strong and intense that I didn't know how to handle them at first.

I realize now that I was experiencing feelings in the way that they are supposed to be felt. Most people cry at movies sometimes, or feel anxious when they have a big exam coming up. These were perfectly *natural* and *normal* reactions to the events in my life. It was just that the antidepressants had caused me to feel these emotions on a much more superficial level. So when I didn't have the drugs to act as a buffer between me and my moods, it felt as though my feelings were much more intense than they really were.

Over time I've realized that it's ok to allow myself to feel. I can get sad when I break up with someone, or angry when I fight with a friend, or nervous when I have to speak in front of a group of people – and this is *completely ok*. Now I must reiterate that if you ever feel so low that you consider harming yourself or someone else, please get help – immediately. Call your doctor or call a friend, and consider going back on antidepressants for the time being. But if you're just having a bad day, and you feel anxious or sad, realize that *everyone* has bad days, and this *doesn't* mean you have an anxiety disorder or depression.

Since I got off antidepressants, I've been through some major stressors in my life. I defended my Ph.D. thesis, and I experienced the sudden and tragic death of my stepfather. When these events happened, I experienced intense emotions. I stood in the washroom at my university before my Ph.D. defense and did my best to calm my shaking hands. I sprawled out on my living room floor after my stepfather died and cried myself to sleep. But I also realized during these times that it was *normal* to feel how I was feeling, and I gave myself permission to let the feelings in.

Everyone needs to have a good cry every once and awhile, especially when they experience tragedy. Believe it or not, crying actually feels good! You know what I'm talking about – that subtle feeling of relief that you get after bawling your eyes out. You're tired, your nose is stuffed up, and you just want to curl up on the couch with a blanket, but you also feel a sense of release.

Let your post-antidepressant feelings in. Don't be scared – feelings won't hurt you. Working through our feelings is what helps us experience personal growth. Use the social support gathered in Chapter 1 to help you through your feelings. Talk to your therapist, talk to a friend, talk to a random stranger in a chat room – just make sure you don't keep pushing your emotions down, because your feelings will ultimately set you free.

Kicking Your Antidepressant Habit Once and For All

I'm here to tell you that you *can* kick your antidepressant habit. It might not be easy, and it might force you to deal with some uncomfortable feelings – feelings that you've kept hidden for a long time, even from yourself. But you can do it. Gradually pull off the antidepressant band aid and give your wounds some air. They need oxygen to heal properly once and for all.

List of Resources

- *"Prozac Backlash"* by Joseph Glenmullen, M.D.
- *"The Antidepressant Solution"* by Joseph Glenmullen, M.D.
- Daily checklist of antidepressant withdrawal symptoms available at: <u>www.drglenmullen.com/AS Appendix 1.pdf</u>.

Chapter 3
Step 3 – Let Go

*I*t was a cold and dreary November evening. After a tough day of working on my thesis, all I wanted to do was go home, curl up in front of the TV, and veg out. Even better, I wanted to engage in my usual practice of ruminating in front of my day planner. This involved creating lists of what I was going to get done each day for the next week, then scanning the lists over and over to make myself feel like I had my schedule under control. This process was not something I enjoyed, but it was a compulsion that I had a hard time ignoring. Unfortunately, I couldn't spend time with my TV or my day planner that evening because I'd promised myself that I would go to yoga. Even more unfortunate was the fact that yoga was the last thing I felt like doing. Mustering all my willpower, I dragged myself to the class. At the studio, I mentally reviewed my task list for the next day while I unrolled my yoga mat. The teacher *entered the room with a soft smile on her face. "Isn't this rain great?" she asked as she breathed in deeply from the studio's open windows. "Mother nature always knows when to give us rain to remind us to take time to turn inward." I stared out at the dismal sky and figured she must have taken drugs before the class. How could she be so content – even happy – about this miserable day?*

~   ~   ~

If you think for a moment about what tends to make you anxious or depressed, you'll probably notice an interesting pattern. When we get anxious, we're often worried about events that might happen in the *future*. When we get depressed, we tend to be sad about events that have happened in the *past*. The unfortunate part about both of these states of thinking is that they prevent us from being in the *now*, in the present moment.

Feelings of anxiety are actually beneficial to humans from an evolutionary perspective. The physiological changes that happen in our body when we get anxious, known as the fight or flight response, help prepare us for danger. Our heart rate speeds up, our breathing becomes shallow, we sweat, the blood flow to our organs and extremities decreases, and our digestive system slows down. This response is exactly what's required to prepare us to fight or flee in a dangerous situation. This built-in response to danger was beneficial millions of years ago when humans spent their days hunting and watching out for saber-toothed tigers. The reason our fight or flight response exists today is that our ancestors who *weren't* hyper-vigilant to danger typically didn't get a chance to pass their genes along to us, because they often got eaten by the saber-toothed tigers.

The problem with the fight or flight response in modern-day humans is that we are no longer faced with the same types of danger that were such a big part of our lives millions of years ago. Another problem is that in humans, the fight or flight response can be triggered by *imagined* fears and anxieties. In other words, you can trigger a stress response in your body by simply *imagining* an anxiety-provoking event that hasn't occurred yet, and that might never occur.

The opposite reaction to fight or flight is the relaxation response, which is a physiological mechanism that helps bring our body back into balance after we experience stress. During the relaxation response, our heart rate stabilizes, our blood pressure evens out, our brain waves slow down, our digestion returns to normal, and we experience a sense of well-being.

A very effective way to reduce anxiety and depression and to stimulate the relaxation response is to engage in practices that help bring us into the present moment. By simply noticing what's happening right now, whether it's good or bad, and not judging it, we diminish our tendency to get worried about things that might happen down the road, or sad about things that have already happened that we can't change.

If I wanted to make this chapter very short, I could sum up my main message as follows: to reduce anxiety and depression, and get off antidepressants, let go of the past and future by focusing only on the present moment. However, I need to make this chapter a little longer, because bringing our attention into the present moment is quite difficult for most people.

Our minds are like an unruly puppy, bouncing from one topic to the next in a never-ending melodrama starring ourselves. In fact, as Marci Shimoff points out in her book *"Happy for No Reason: 7 Steps to Being Happy from the Inside Out,"* studies have shown that the average person has around 60,000 thoughts per day – which is one thought per second for every hour that we're awake! Interestingly, 95% of these thoughts are the same thoughts we had yesterday and the day before. The most unfortunate part of this statistic is that 80%, or 45,000 of our 60,000 daily thoughts are *negative*. In other words, we tend to think the same negative thoughts over and over again.

How can you possibly get off antidepressants amidst all these negative thoughts? By continually bringing your attention into the present moment and letting go of your thoughts. Three techniques that have been absolutely crucial in helping me come into the present moment are meditation, yoga, and breathwork.

Meditation

It's been a hard day at work. I come home, sit on my yoga mat, and decide to spend some time meditating. I begin by focusing on my breath as it comes in and out of my nose. I gradually slow my inhalations and exhalations and begin to feel the tension draining from my body. Just as I'm starting to let go, I think to myself, "Wow, I'm meditating really well today! I thought I would have trouble meditating because of the tough day I had at work, but I'm doing great! Speaking of work, I wonder if I'll be able to get that report done by Friday. Man, they've really been pushing us with deadlines lately. I think that's why my shoulders are so tight. Speaking of my shoulders, I wish the sunburn on my back would stop peeling. Maybe I should rub some cream on it after I finish meditating. Oh yeah – I'm supposed to be meditating! Now I've wrecked the great meditation practice that I started. I was doing so well and now it's ruined. Why can't I meditate properly?"

~   ~   ~

The practice of meditation has existed for thousands of years, and can be done in a multitude of ways. My purpose here is to outline a few meditation concepts and techniques that have worked for me. The story above is typical of what happens to many people when they begin meditating. But as I will describe below, there really is no right or wrong way to meditate. So don't place too much pressure on yourself to meditate "properly!" If your mind is busy or preoccupied, your meditation hasn't been ruined, because you can always bring your attention back into the present moment.

For those who would like a more in-depth explanation of some of the concepts that I describe below, I strongly suggest the books *"A Gradual Awakening"* by Stephen Levine, *"Wherever You Go, There You Are"* by Jon Kabat-Zinn, and *"The Power of Now"* by Eckhart Tolle.

What is Meditation?

At its very core, meditation involves taking some time to quiet your mind and come into the present moment. This can be done in an enormous number of ways – you can meditate while sitting, laying down, or walking. You can meditate by staring at a candle, or with your eyes closed. You can meditate by focusing on a picture, a word, or a sentence, or even by focusing on the sensations in your body. Meditation, in its variety of forms, has been practiced by people from all walks of life and spiritual traditions for millennia.

The topic of meditation makes some people uneasy because they think that to meditate they will have to join some far off religious cult. One thing that I want to make very clear is that meditation is *not* a religion. People from all sorts of spiritual backgrounds, from Catholics to Hindus to Muslims, often practice some form of meditation, whether it's through prayer or a more formal meditation practice. You don't need to be spiritual or religious to meditate. You also don't have to live on a mountain in the Himalayas or join an ashram. Meditation can be done anywhere – in your home, in your office, or even in your car!

One form of meditation that I've found particularly helpful in relieving my anxiety and sadness is mindfulness meditation. Mindfulness meditation uses various techniques to bring your attention into the present moment. In his book *"Wherever You Go, There You Are,"* Jon Kabat-Zinn describes mindfulness as:

> *"...paying attention in a particular way: on purpose, in the present moment, and non-judgmentally. This kind of attention nurtures greater awareness, clarity, and acceptance of present-moment reality. It wakes us up to the fact that our lives unfold only in moments. If we are not fully present for many of those moments, we may not only miss what is most valuable in our lives but also fail to realize the richness and the depth of our possibilities for growth and transformation."*

There is a profound truth in the practice of mindfulness – the present moment is all we have. The past is finished, and we never know for certain what the future holds. We could die at any moment, which makes our worries about the future a futile exercise. Bringing our attention into the present and simply witnessing what's happening, without labeling it as good or bad, allows us to calm our anxiety and quell our sadness.

A large body of research exists on the beneficial physical and mental effects of meditation. Neuroscientists have repeatedly found that the brains of people who meditate regularly are both structurally and functionally different from the brains of people who don't meditate. As an example, studies have shown that meditation is linked to healthy changes in areas of the brain that are responsible for emotional processing and well-being. Meditators also show increased activity in the areas of their brain that are associated with positive emotions and concentration. Meditation has even been found to alleviate the symptoms associated with migraines and asthma, as well as chronic pain, high blood pressure, heart disease, anxiety, depression, and cancer.

Research has confirmed over and over that meditation is beneficial for a myriad of conditions. Meditation represents a natural and effective way to help you reduce anxiety and depression without having to depend on antidepressant medication.

Mindfulness Meditation Techniques

There are several techniques that you can use to bring your attention into the present moment. I outline just a few of them here.

Focusing on the Body and/or Breath

One of the first forms of mindfulness meditation that I learned was to come into the present by focusing on my breathing. You can do this sitting up or lying down, with your eyes open and unfocused or closed. Start by getting into a position that's comfortable for you, and begin bringing your attention to how your breath feels as it comes in and out of your nose. Don't judge your breath or try to change it. Just observe how it feels on your upper lip every time you breathe in and out.

While you're focusing on your breath, thoughts are going to come into your mind. Try to become an unbiased observer of your thoughts. As best you can, try to watch the thoughts pass by like you're watching the closing credits on a movie screen. Avoid engaging in a conversation with your thoughts. Every time your mind veers off, notice that this has happened and return your attention to your breath.

As an example, if you suddenly have the thought "I need to get groceries tonight," avoid elaborating on this thought with more thoughts like "…I think we need green peppers, but I'm not sure – did I buy some last week? I don't like the green peppers at the market down the road. I wonder where they get their produce. It used to be so good..." If this type of internal dialogue starts to happen, don't get upset with yourself. Simply notice your thoughts and then return to the breath. If it's helpful, you can even label your thoughts. Every time a thought comes to mind, simply say the word "thought" to yourself, and return your attention to your breath.

If focusing on your breath feels strange to you, try focusing on your bodily sensations instead. The process is exactly the same as what I've described above, except instead of bringing your attention back to the breath every time your mind veers off, you bring it back to your body. Notice how your muscles feel. Notice the temperature of the room on your skin. You can choose to focus on one specific part of your body, like your stomach or your hands, or you can do "body scans" by moving your awareness from your head to your feet over and over again.

If there's a part of your body that's in pain or uncomfortable, you can bring your attention there and simply focus on that area – without judging it or trying to make the pain go away. Remarkably, this focus can help relieve the pain. In his book *"Full Catastrophe Living: Using the Wisdom of Your Body and Mind to Face Stress, Pain, and Illness,"* Jon Kabat-Zinn goes into great detail about the ways in which mindfulness meditation can help relieve chronic pain.

Focusing on a Candle or Picture

You can also practice mindfulness meditation by focusing on an external object. This can be particularly helpful if you suffer from panic attacks that are exacerbated when you focus too closely on your bodily sensations. Try lighting a candle and gazing at it, allowing your eyes to become unfocused while you meditate. As thoughts enter your mind, simply bring your attention back to the candle. You can also focus on a picture to meditate. You can choose a picture that's particularly meaningful to you, or use a mandala. Mandala is a Sanskrit word that means "circle." True to their name, mandalas are circular images that often contain intricate designs. These pictures can help you focus while you meditate.

Focusing on a Mantra

A mantra is a word or sentence that you repeat to yourself to focus your attention while you meditate. You can choose any word or sentence that works well for you. For example, you might want to repeat the words "All is well," or "I am at peace," or "Love." Another helpful mantra involves repeating the words "I am breathing in, I am breathing out."

To focus your attention and keep your mind from drifting, you can use mala beads while you repeat your mantra. A mala necklace or bracelet is made up of a string of 108 beads. A mala has 108 beads because this number is considered to be auspicious and sacred in many Eastern cultures. Similar to a rosary in the Catholic faith, you hold your mala and recite your mantra 108 times – once for each bead. Noticing how each bead feels between your fingers as you meditate is a great way to keep your mind in the present moment by giving you some tactile stimulation to focus on.

Focusing on Your Movement

If you find sitting still difficult, you can also practice mindfulness meditation while you walk. To do so, find a place where you can walk slowly without being disturbed. Many people who practice walking meditation walk in a circle, with their hands behind their back as they gaze downward at their feet. If you feel like you might look silly doing this, try practicing walking meditation in a private place like your backyard, or even in a large room in your house.

Walking meditation can be done when you're trying to get somewhere, but it's often nice to practice this form of meditation by walking in a circle without having anywhere to go. Either way, the point is to walk slowly and purposefully, focusing on how each step feels in your body. Every time your mind drifts, you bring your attention back to your feet. You can also combine walking meditation with a mantra, such as "One foot in front of the other."

Bringing Your Attention into the Present

All the forms of meditation described above accomplish the same goal – they help us decrease anxiety about the future and depression about the past by bringing our attention into the present. Practicing mindfulness meditation doesn't mean you have to get rid of all your thoughts – it means you notice your thoughts and avoid reacting to them. Mindfulness also doesn't equate to never planning for the future or eliminating your memories. Sometimes you have to plan for events that are coming down the road, or remember something that happened to you.

The basic idea behind meditation is that as you increasingly allow yourself to be in the moment, you can prepare for the future from a clearer and calmer place. For example, if I need to plan what I'll be doing tomorrow, I can start by focusing on my breath and calming my mind. Then, I do only the amount of planning necessary for tomorrow. When I'm done, I let that planning go and I come back into the present.

Different forms of meditation work best for different people. Try a few techniques and see what works for you. And try to reserve your judgments about whether you're meditating "properly." In meditation, there's nothing to attain. Your meditation practice is neither good, nor bad. It just is. As Jon Kabat-Zinn often says, "If the mind wanders off a thousand times, you simply bring it back a thousand times." Some days your mind will be extremely busy. This doesn't make you a "bad meditator." If you start thinking you're a bad meditator while you're meditating, just notice these thoughts, and then return your attention to the present.

If meditation is new to you, start small. Don't suddenly expect yourself to be able to meditate for an hour every day. Even 5 minutes a day is a step in the right direction. If you can't commit to a daily practice, try every other day, or even once a week. Over time, you'll start to crave meditation as you begin to experience its beneficial effects.

If you're interested in buying CDs or MP3s that will guide you through a mindfulness meditation practice, I recommend Jon Kabat-Zinn's Series 2 *"Guided Mindfulness Meditation"* CDs, which are available at www. mindfulnesscds.com. Jon Kabat-Zinn also has several guided meditations available at www.amazon.com and through iTunes.

Yoga

I walk into my first advanced yoga class with butterflies in my stomach. All of the students in the class, including myself, are yoga teachers in training. Despite the fact that I've been practicing yoga for several years, I feel apprehensive about the class. Several students are "warming up" with headstands and handstands, while I can barely touch my toes!

I take a deep breath and sit on my mat. The teacher enters the room and starts off with a few gentle stretches. As I move and breathe, I begin to experience a feeling that comes on like an old familiar friend. It's the feeling of releasing tension from my body and mind. Everything becomes softer – my muscles, my thoughts, and my emotions. I gradually bring my attention inward and focus only on myself, as if I'm the only student in the class.

As the teacher begins demonstrating the advanced poses, I calmly do only what my body can handle. Each student in the class is like a unique beam of light, with both strengths and weaknesses. I give up the need to compare myself to others, and open myself to the learning being provided by the teacher.

At the end of the class, as we all lay on our backs in corpse pose, it's as if our beams of light join together, surrounding us with a warm, beautiful energy. Through our practice, we've calmed our bodies and minds, let go of what no longer serves us, and supported each other's learning. A small smile comes to my lips as I realize that each yoga class, no matter how easy or difficult, serves as a constant reminder of why I continue to practice.

~   ~   ~

What is Yoga?

The practice of yoga is ancient, with its historical roots dating back to 3000 B.C. The word "yoga" is derived from the word "*yuj*", which means yoke, union, or connection. The ultimate goal of yoga is to join the individual self with the larger, infinite, universal self. In essence, yoga helps bring us back to our true nature, which is peaceful and full of joy.

In the Western world, yoga is often associated with physical postures that are done in a studio or gym. However, yoga also has a vast philosophical and spiritual component that can be adopted if one chooses. Similar to meditation, yoga is not a religion, and you don't need to be spiritual or religious to practice yoga. You can choose to explore the spiritual aspects of yoga, or you can simply do physical yoga postures for their stress-relieving benefits. Either way, yoga is an essential tool in your quest toward antidepressant freedom.

Over the past three decades, research on the beneficial physical and mental effects of yoga has steadily grown. Yoga activates our body's natural capacity to heal itself, and has been found to improve mood, reduce stress, and boost our immune system. Yoga has also been found to alleviate the symptoms of cardiovascular disease, respiratory disorders like asthma, endocrine disorders like diabetes, and several neurological conditions. Yoga benefits all our bodily systems, including our bones, muscles, circulation, respiration, digestion, endocrine system, and nervous system. Yoga also helps the brain release serotonin.

One very important thing to keep in mind is that you don't need to be able to twist yourself into a pretzel to go to a yoga class. I'm a certified yoga teacher with over 200 hours of yoga training, and I can't even touch my toes! I strongly believe that yoga can be done by people of all shapes, ages, sizes, and levels of flexibility. Sure, you might need to modify the poses slightly to meet your needs, but you can still do yoga.

Types of Yoga

Many, many different types of yoga exist. Some yoga teachers subscribe to only one tradition, while other teachers combine aspects of multiple traditions to provide an eclectic approach. For example, I was trained by teachers who came from the Kripalu tradition, however even as I was doing my training these teachers were exploring Anusara yoga. This is why it's important to "shop around" until you find a teacher and a style of yoga that works for you. Every teacher is different!

Below I describe a few of common types of yoga. This list is by no means exhaustive, but it will help give you an idea of the variety of styles of yoga that are out there.

- **Kripalu Yoga** focuses on physical postures, as well as psychological growth and spiritual awakening. Kripalu teachers focus on body alignment, breathing techniques, surrendering into the postures, and trusting the natural intelligence of the body to move and heal itself. For more information, visit www.kripalu.org.

- **Iyengar Yoga** focuses on the subtle muscular and skeletal alignment of each yoga pose. Postures are often held for longer than in other forms of yoga so that the student can experience each pose at a very deep level. Props such as blocks, straps, and blankets are often used to modify the poses to accommodate individual needs. For more information, visit www.iyisf.org.

- **Kundalini Yoga** incorporates physical postures, breathing techniques, chanting, and meditation to move energy upward from the base of the spine. Practitioners of this style of yoga believe that we each hold powerful energy that is coiled like a serpent at the base of our spine. Moving this energy upward through the body's major energy centers is believed to eventually lead to an enlightened state. For more information, visit www.3HO.org.

- **Bikram Yoga** is also known as hot yoga or Moksha yoga. A typical class includes a series of 26 postures that are done in a very hot room, with temperatures of up to 100 degrees Fahrenheit. Sweat is believed to detoxify the body, while the heat helps improve flexibility. For more information, visit www.bikramyoga. com.

- **Anusara Yoga** focuses on aligning the physical and mental body by integrating body alignment with opening the heart (both physically and emotionally). The Anusara philosophy holds that we are all divine and perfect, and aims to help people re-discover their true nature. For more information, visit www.anusara.com.
- **Ashtanga Yoga**. The form of Ashtanga yoga that has been popularized in the West is quite physical and vigorous. It includes six series of postures that increase in difficulty and are done at a fast pace. If you need a boost in energy and are prepared to sweat, this style of yoga could work for you. For more information, visit www. ashtanga.com.
- **Power Yoga**. As its name suggests, power yoga is vigorous and develops strength and flexibility. Students are often asked to move from pose to pose quickly, so that the poses make up a series of flowing movements also known as a vinyasa. For more information, visit www.poweryoga.com.
- **Restorative Yoga** is meant to be extremely calming and rejuvenating. It involves adapting classic yoga postures by using props like

blankets and cushions, so that the student is *passively* supported in the pose. The poses are held for longer than in a typical yoga class, but the postures don't require a large exertion of energy. This allows the student to focus on releasing tension and brings the body and mind back into balance. For more information, see the book *"Relax and Renew"* by Judith Lasater.

- **Hatha Yoga**. This is a term that is often used to describe a combination of several forms of yoga. If a class or DVD is described as Hatha Yoga, try to find out the level of intensity that will be required for the class so that you can decide if it would be right for you.

What Type of Yoga is Right for You?

I guarantee that if you look hard enough, you will find a style of yoga that suits your needs. If you try a certain teacher or studio that doesn't feel right, try something else. Eventually you will find a style of yoga that matches who you are and that helps you along in your journey.

Different styles of yoga might work better for you depending on whether you suffer predominantly from depression versus anxiety. If you suffer from depression, it's often a good idea to do a slightly more vigorous yoga class that will help you increase your energy. If you tend to be anxious, it's best to find a gentle class that will help you slow down and move inward. I've tried several forms of yoga over the years, including Bikram, Kripalu, Kundalini, Power Yoga, Anusara Yoga, and Restorative Yoga. Each type of yoga was beneficial in its own way, depending on what I needed at the time.

I will say, however, that Restorative Yoga was *extremely* effective at helping me reduce my anxiety. Being a high-strung, Type A person, I was often drawn to yoga classes that were vigorous and intense. After trying restorative yoga, I realized that what I really needed to do was slow down. Restorative yoga wasn't easy for me at first, as it mostly involves laying still and focusing on the breath. I have a hard time staying still, and I was dying to get up and move! But I stuck with restorative yoga, and the results were amazing. I credit restorative yoga as one of the main factors that helped me reduce my anxiety to a point where I could live without antidepressants.

In the end, you will probably need to try a few different styles of yoga and yoga teachers before you find one that's exactly right for you. But please don't give up. Yoga can keep you off antidepressants over the long term by helping you manage your anxiety and mood.

Yoga Postures

Yoga postures operate at a very subtle level. These poses not only increase our flexibility, calm us, and give us energy – they also enhance our awareness of the intimate connection between our physical bodies and our minds.

In essence, yoga teaches us that our bodies are the physical manifestation of our minds. When you feel anxious or depressed, your body often develops physical symptoms associated with these feelings, such as tight shoulders, stomach upset, or weight gain. Take a moment right now to slump your shoulders forward and put a frown on your face. Notice how this makes you feel. Now sit up tall, open your arms wide, take a deep breath, and smile. Notice a difference? These two postures evoke very different emotions and physiological reactions in our bodies.

Similarly, yoga postures help us release emotional manifestations from our body by changing not only our physiology but also our energy. Some yoga postures expand, open, and energize our bodies, while others calm and soothe. This is why different types of yoga work best for different people. While practicing yoga poses, it's helpful to also practice mindfulness. Come into the moment and notice how each pose makes you feel, both physically and mentally.

There are hundreds of yoga postures in existence, which makes it impossible to describe them all here. For those who are interested in learning more about yoga poses, I recommend the book *"Yoga Mind, Body, and Spirit"* by Donna Farhi, as well as the website www.

<u>yogajournal.com</u> (click on the "poses" tab at the top of the page to see pictures of all sorts of yoga poses).

<u>Philosophical Components of Yoga</u>

In the third century B.C., a sage named Patanjali produced four books called the Yoga Sutras. These four books are comprised of a series of 196 verses that describe the entire philosophy of yoga. The Yoga Sutras also provide clear techniques to reach the ultimate goals of yoga, which are physical health, mental awareness and harmony, and a return to our true self by experiencing the union of our inner spirit with the universal spirit.

In the Yoga Sutras, Patanjali outlines an eight-limbed path to help practitioners attain these goals. This path contains tips and techniques that are just as applicable today as they were thousands of years ago. I briefly describe the eight-limbed path here. Those who are interested in learning more about yoga philosophy and the eight-limbed path are encouraged to read *"Yoga Mind, Body, and Spirit"* by Donna Farhi, *"Yoga and the Quest for the True Self"* by Stephen Cope, and *"The Inner Tradition of Yoga: A Guide to Yoga Philosophy for the Contemporary Practitioner"* by Michael Stone.

The eight limbs of yoga include:

1. **The Yamas**. The five *Yamas* are moral principles that advise us on how to best use our energy in relation to others and ourselves:

- *Ahimsa*, or nonviolence, involves having compassion for all living things, including ourselves.
- *Satya*, or truthfulness, involves being truthful in all of our actions.
- *Asteya*, or nonstealing, goes beyond the simple idea of not shoplifting. *Asteya* also asks us to avoid taking that which has not been freely given to us, whether this is a material possession or someone's time and energy.
- *Brahmacarya*, or moderation, asks us to avoid overindulging and urges us to relax into our lives by believing that we are guided and supported by a higher power.
- *Aparigraha*, or nongrasping, asks us to live in simplicity by releasing our attachment to material possessions and letting go of our need to always be in control.
2. **The Niyamas**. The five *Niyamas* give us a code for ethical living and relate to the choices that we make in our lives:
- *Sauca*, or purity, involves keeping our minds, bodies, and environments clean to avoid confusion and chaos in our lives.
- *Santosa*, or contentment, involves accepting what is, being satisfied with whatever is happening in the present moment, and making the best out of every situation.

- *Tapas*, or burning enthusiasm, involves having the energy and discipline to do what's necessary to meet our goals.
- *Svadhyaya*, or self-study, involves engaging in activities that help us learn about and understand ourselves. The activity itself could be anything, such as reading, journaling, or even playing sports – as long as it helps us engage in self-reflection.
- *Isvara-pranidhana*, or celebration of the spiritual, involves surrendering to a higher power and taking time to recognize that there is a force larger than ourselves that's directing our lives.

3. **Asana**, or yoga postures, allow us to develop strength, flexibility, and a relaxed body so that we can strengthen the connection between the physical and mental aspects of ourselves. In the West, we tend to focus most on this aspect of the eight-limbed path. However, it's important to remember that physical postures are only one part of the larger philosophy of yoga.

4. **Pranayama**, or mindful breathing practices, help us move our prana, or life force, to promote relaxation, remove energy blockages in our bodies, and increase our vitality. I cover breathing practices in more detail in the next section.

5. **Pratyahara**, or turning inward, involves turning our attention toward stillness as opposed to over-stimulating the senses with things like loud music or TV.

6. **Dharana**, or concentration, involves focusing our attention on a single mental object, thereby taking our attention away from the distractions of the mind.

7. **Dhyana**, or meditation, involves bringing our attention into the present moment and sustaining our awareness regardless of what's going on around us. Dhyana is different from Dharana in that in Dhyana, we sustain our awareness without the need to focus on a mental object. Dhyana is a state of stillness with few or no thoughts at all.

8. **Samadhi**, or enlightenment, involves a complete union of the self with all other living things. Samadhi is an experience of bliss and oneness with the universe. It is the experience of true inner peace.

Over the centuries, some have viewed this eight-limbed path as a hierarchical progression that should be followed from step 1 to 8 to reach enlightenment. However many people, including myself, prefer to see the eight-limbed path as the spokes of a wheel, or as a spiral. The eight spokes or components of the spiral can be practiced in any order, because each component influences each other component. For example, if you begin with the practice of *Dhyana* (meditation), you will probably eventually be drawn toward *Asana* (yoga postures). If you begin with *Asana*, you will likely be drawn at some point to ethical living through the *Yamas* and *Niyamas*.

In sum, practicing yoga helps reduce your need for antidepressants by releasing tension in your mind and body, and by helping you move toward a life of stillness and peace. Begin practicing yoga regularly and I guarantee you will notice a change in both your mental and physical health.

Breathwork

My stomach is bunched up in a tight knot. I have so much to do that I don't even know where to start. Should I work on my thesis? Or should I start preparing for the lecture that I need to present tomorrow? Oh wait – I also need to run a few errands and I'm supposed to make dinner tonight. My mind races with what seems like 50 million thoughts at once. My chest moves frantically up and down while I take short, quick gasps of air. It feels like I have no control over my pounding heart, and I'm beginning to feel sharp pains in my abdomen. These stomach pains are all too familiar – I half-jokingly call them my "ulcer pains" as they seem to appear whenever I get anxious.

Suddenly, for a fraction of a second, I come into the present moment. I notice how shallow my breathing has become. I very gently start to slow my breathing down, bringing my breath all the way down into my belly. I deliberately alter my breathing pattern to make it slower and deeper. After a few moments, my heart rate slows down, and my mind begins to clear. The knot in my belly starts to unravel, and the pain in my abdomen slowly dissipates. After only a few minutes of adjusting my breathing, I feel composed and rejuvenated.

~   ~   ~

What is Breathwork?

I want to focus on breathwork, or *Pranayama*, in more detail for a moment, because changing the way I breathed was absolutely essential to helping me get off, and stay off, antidepressants. When we feel anxious, we tend to breathe shallowly from our upper chest. You've probably had this experience before – you begin to feel anxious and you start to take short, gasping breaths. This type of breathing can even turn into hyperventilation in some cases.

As adults, we often become so accustomed to breathing shallowly that we aren't even aware that our natural state involves breathing much more deeply. Have you ever watched a baby's belly while it breathes? Innocent and unconditioned by the stressors of adult life, babies breathe fully and deeply from their diaphragm. Their belly moves outward and expands when they inhale, and contracts when they exhale. One very effective way to reduce anxiety and depression as adults is to remind our bodies how to breathe in this natural and relaxed way.

Our breath is intimately connected to our nervous system. When we take short breaths from our upper chest, our bodies release a flood of chemicals that prepare us for danger. When we breathe slowly and deeply, we send signals to our body that we are relaxed and at ease. Our breath is the only physiological function in our bodies that is controlled by both our voluntary and involuntary nervous system. In other words, you don't have to tell yourself to breathe in and out – this happens involuntarily. But you can also voluntarily *change* your breathing pattern to promote a more relaxed state.

Changing our breathing patterns to promote relaxation can have profoundly beneficial effects on our digestion, circulation, immune and endocrine systems. Regulating the breath can also help you reduce blood pressure, slow your heart rate, lower your stress hormones, and even release neurotransmitters like serotonin. Importantly, the way that we breathe directly influences our mind. Harnessing the power of the breath to naturally reduce anxiety and depression is an extremely powerful way to avoid depending on antidepressants to alter your mood.

Breathing Exercises

Below I give a brief description of seven breathing techniques that, if practiced regularly, are guaranteed to reduce your anxiety and depression. For those who are interested in learning more about the power of the breath, I recommend "*The Breathing Book*" by Donna Farhi.

Each of the breathing techniques below can be done anytime, anywhere to help reduce anxiety when you're stressed or increase your energy when you feel low. Before beginning each technique, start by taking a few normal breaths to establish a steady rhythm. Unless otherwise noted, all of these breathing techniques involve inhaling and exhaling through your nose, not your mouth. If you feel anxious or short of breath at any point while practicing these exercises, simply return to your natural breathing pattern and then try again. I've listed the techniques in sequential order – so it's important to master the techniques at the beginning of the list before you move forward.

Extended Exhalation

Begin by simply observing the feeling of your breath as it comes in and out of your nose. When you feel ready, gently draw your abdominal muscles back as you come to the end of your exhalation, allowing your exhalation to be one or two counts longer than your inhalation. Then inhale naturally and repeat the process. For example, if your inhalation lasts five seconds, allow your exhalation to last seven seconds. Then inhale for five seconds, exhale for seven seconds, and so forth. This breathing technique is very calming for the nervous system, and can be practiced to reduce tension when you feel stressed.

Three-Part Breathing (Dirgha Breath)

This breathing technique involves filling all three chambers of the lungs, beginning with the lower abdomen, then moving up to the mid-chest region, and ending in the upper chest. As you inhale, gently bring your breath down into your belly. Your belly will move outward as it expands. As you continue to inhale, bring your breath into your mid-chest and then upper chest. Exhale slowly, releasing the breath first from the belly, then mid-chest, then upper chest. Try not to force your belly to move outward or to contract – even if your belly only moves a little bit, this is ok. Continue taking long, smooth breaths in this way. This breathing technique is calming, detoxifying, and rejuvenating.

Breath of Victory (Ujjayi Breath)

Begin by taking long, slow, deep breaths through the nostrils. When you're ready, narrow the back of your throat slightly to create a hissing sound that resembles the rise and fall of ocean waves (or Darth Vader!). Create this sound on both the inhalation and the exhalation.

You can combine this breath with the three-part breath if you would like. This breathing technique is very calming, reduces stress, and increases concentration.

Square or Box Breath

In this breath, you pause at the end of the inhalation and at the end of the exhalation, with the length of all the sections of your breath being the same. The pattern is inhale, pause, exhale, pause. Begin by counting the length of your inhalation, then pause, holding your breath for that same amount of time, then exhale for the same amount of time, then pause for the same amount of time, and so forth. For example, if your inhalation lasts 5 seconds, you would inhale for 5 seconds, pause for 5 seconds, exhale for 5 seconds, pause for 5 seconds, and so forth. This breathing technique is very stabilizing and grounding, and increases your ability to breathe more fully.

Alternate Nostril Breathing

This breathing technique is best done from a seated or standing position (not laying down). Begin with the three-part breath. Inhale, then close your right nostril with your right thumb. Exhale and then inhale through your left nostril. At the end of your inhalation, remove your thumb from your right nostril, and close your left nostril with your index finger. Exhale and then inhale through your right nostril. At the end of your inhalation, release your left nostril and close your right nostril. This completes one cycle. Repeat this cycle for two minutes or longer. This breathing technique is very stabilizing for the nervous system, and helps balance the two hemispheres of our brain. It's also calming, helps improve mental clarity, and heightens concentration.

Skull-Shining Breath (Kapalabathi Breath)

This breathing technique is best done from a seated or standing position (not laying down). Inhale, allowing your belly to expand, then exhale sharply to push the air out through your nose (almost like someone has punched you in the stomach and "knocked the wind" out of you). Allow your next inhalation to be completely passive – your breath will come back in naturally as your abdominal muscles return to their normal position.

Inhale slowly and fully before doing another exhalation – your exhalations should come every 2 to 3 seconds. Repeat for one to three minutes. This breathing technique is detoxifying, energizing, creates mental alertness, and increases your resistance to stress. You shouldn't perform this breathing technique if you're pregnant, have uncontrolled high blood pressure, a hiatal hernia, an abdominal disorder, or any herniated discs. Proceed with caution with this breathing technique if you're menstruating, or if you have any respiratory or cardiovascular conditions.

Bellows Breath (Bhastrika Breath)

This breathing technique is similar to Skull-Shining Breath except that it's done faster, by exhaling at a pace of one breath per second for a minute at a time. Inhale sharply through your nose and expand your belly, then exhale forcefully out of your nose by snapping your belly back toward your spine. Continue this cycle for ten breaths, without pausing between the inhalation and exhalation.

After ten breaths, rest by doing several three-part breaths. If you get light-headed, stop and rest for a few minutes, then try again if you feel comfortable. The same precautions and contraindications exist for this breathing technique as for the Skull-Shining Breath. This breathing technique is very stimulating, increases your resistance to stress, improves mental alertness, and is great when you need a boost of energy.

Taken together, these breathing techniques provide you with several tools that you can use at any time to help reduce your stress and increase your energy. These breathing exercises were crucial in helping me get off antidepressants, and I still use many of them regularly to stabilize my mood.

My Experiences with Meditation, Yoga, and Breathwork

Meditation, yoga, and breathwork were all critical in helping me get off antidepressants. These practices helped me let go, calm my mind, improve the flow of energy in my body, reduce my stress, and increase my happiness. I see these practices as natural and healthy alternatives to antidepressant medication.

One interesting thing that I've noticed about meditation, yoga, and breathwork is that although they are among the *best* practices for me to do; they are often the *hardest* things for me to get myself to do. As I mentioned in the story at the beginning of this chapter, it's much easier for me to sit around and ruminate, or veg out in front of the TV, than to drag myself to a yoga class.

Whenever I used to meet a new yoga teacher, I would think "Wow, I wish I could be like her, so calm and at peace." But the truth is that yoga teachers don't have magical powers. The only difference between them and me was that by practicing yoga regularly, they were making a conscious choice to keep their life in balance. I soon realized that I needed to start making the same types of choices to keep my anxiety and sadness in check.

Meditation, yoga, and breathwork involve a continuing journey that I'm still taking to this day. There are still lots of times when I don't feel like doing yoga. And I definitely don't wake up at 5:30am, bright-eyed and eager to meditate. Sometimes I still have trouble meditating for even 10 minutes at a time – but I do what I can and I let the rest go. As much as possible, I bring myself to my mat and I just start. Even 5, 10, or 15 minutes a day of yoga, meditation, or breathing exercises is better than nothing. You don't need to suddenly become a guru or start doing yoga every day. Start small.

If yoga doesn't appeal to you, try some other form of physical activity, like aerobics, running, tai chi, or karate. Numerous studies have demonstrated the stress-reducing and mood-enhancing effects of regular physical exercise. Moderate-intensity exercise, like jogging, cycling, swimming, or brisk walking for 20-30 minutes, 4 to 5 times per week is all that's needed to experience these mood-enhancing effects. Importantly, exercise can take a couple of months to reach its full antidepressant effect, so don't give up until you've given it a try for at least awhile. And while doing yoga or exercising might not be as easy as popping an antidepressant every day, the results are well worth it.

Nowadays I'm increasingly bringing meditation, yoga, and breathwork into my daily life. For example, when I feel anxious at work, I practice extended exhalations while I sit at my desk. I practice *Pratyahara* (turning inward) by keeping the radio off in my car. I engage in *Ahimsa* (nonviolence) to the earth by trying to recycle more. And I practice mindfulness by standing in the grass in my backyard without my shoes on, focusing on how the earth feels between my toes. For more examples of how to bring yogic principles into your everyday life, check out *"Bringing Yoga to Life: The Everyday Practice of Enlightened Being"* by Donna Farhi.

As you become more experienced on the yogic path, you will notice that the practice of yoga goes far beyond the physical postures. Yoga begins to infiltrate many other areas of your life. As my yoga teachers often say, "It's all yoga." Every experience that you have in life is an opportunity to practice a yogic principle, whether it's mindfulness, moderation, self-discipline, or one of the myriad other principles. As you begin to exist more and more in the present moment, you will gradually let go of the need for antidepressants, because there's nothing to be anxious or sad about. All you have is this moment, right here, right now, and it's absolutely perfect as it is.

List of Resources

- *"Happy for No Reason: 7 Steps to Being Happy from the Inside Out"* by Marci Shimoff.
- *"A Gradual Awakening"* by Stephen Levine.
- *"Wherever You Go, There You Are"* by Jon Kabat-Zinn.
- *"The Power of Now"* by Eckhart Tolle.
- *"Full Catastrophe Living: Using the Wisdom of Your Body and Mind to Face Stress, Pain, and Illness"* by Jon Kabat-Zinn.
- Jon Kabat-Zinn's Series 2 *"Guided Mindfulness Meditation"* CDs, which are available at www.mindfulnesscds.com.
- Kripalu yoga: www.kripalu.org.
- Iyengar yoga: www.iyisf.org.
- Kundalini yoga: www.3HO.org.
- Bikram yoga: www.bikramyoga.com.
- Anusara yoga: www.anusara.com.
- Ashtanga yoga: www.ashtanga.com.
- Power yoga: www.poweryoga.com.
- Restorative yoga: See the book *"Relax and Renew"* by Judith Lasater.
- *"Yoga Mind, Body, and Spirit"* by Donna Farhi
- Yoga poses: www.yogajournal.com (click on the "poses" tab at the top of the page to see pictures of all sorts of yoga poses).

- *"Yoga and the Quest for the True Self"* by Stephen Cope.
- *"The Inner Tradition of Yoga: A Guide to Yoga Philosophy for the Contemporary Practitioner"* by Michael Stone.
- *"The Breathing Book"* by Donna Farhi.
- *"Bringing Yoga to Life: The Everyday Practice of Enlightened Being"* by Donna Farhi.

Chapter 4
Step 4 – Choose Wisely

*I*t's a Tuesday just like any other Tuesday. I wake up at 7am, do my morning routine, and get in the car to go to work. I pull out of the driveway and wave good-bye to my husband. Then, right on cue at around 8:15am, my eyes well up with tears. I take a deep breath and fight against the sadness in my heart. I don't want to go to work. It's not that I hate my job – it pays well and I enjoy the company of my co-workers – but it isn't what I'm truly meant to do. Plus, I've been working a ton of overtime, I'm exhausted, and I'm having all sorts of vague health problems that my doctor can't figure out.

I grip the steering wheel as a sharp pain rips through my belly. My stomach has been hurting a lot over the past week, but I have so much work to do that there's no way I can take a sick day. I pull into the parking lot and drag my feet to my cubicle. I sit at my desk and take another deep breath as my stomach reels with pain. As I look at *my calendar to assess the day ahead, something in my brain clicks.*

I can't do this anymore.

I can no longer live a life that denies my soul's true purpose. I can no longer ignore my body's physical signs that are screaming at me. On the one hand, I'm doing everything that society tells me I'm supposed to do. I have a Ph.D., a good job, a loving husband, a house, and a car. I want for nothing – except to get my life back. While it looks good on paper, my job is robbing me of my livelihood.

On that ordinary Tuesday morning, I stood up, grabbed my bag, and walked out of the office. When I got home, I wrote my boss an email asking for a sick day, and fell into bed to have a big long cry. Deep down inside, I knew I wasn't going back.

~   ~   ~

I believe that when it comes to living the life we truly want, we almost *always* have a choice in the matter. Even in situations where we feel completely stuck and helpless, there is often a perspective that we haven't considered that will bring us one step closer to fulfillment.

Now when I say we have a choice, I'm not implying that this choice is easy. On the contrary, it's often much easier for us to stick with the status quo of our current jobs, relationships, and habits, than to make the sometimes tough choices that will move us toward antidepressant freedom. To get rid of the personal and professional shackles that can chain us to antidepressants, we often have to make difficult decisions.

In her book *"Happy for No Reason"* Marci Shimoff suggests that everything we do in life either expands our energy or contracts it. Think about the things that make you happy – truly blissful and content, like having dinner with a loved one or spending a day on the beach. Notice how your energy feels – open, expansive, and joyful. Now think of something that's frustrating or making you sad. Notice the difference in your energy – tight, anxious, heavy.

Make a list of the things in your life that expand your energy versus contract it. What you'll probably notice is that you have at least some degree of control over many of the things that are contracting your energy. However, we're often so stuck in our limited patterns of thinking that we fail to see the ways that we could make our lives better. Or we're too scared to take an uncharted path that might ultimately enhance our well-being, because the uncharted path isn't what society thinks we should do.

In Chapter 3 I mentioned the fact that 95% of the thoughts that you have today are the same as the thoughts you had yesterday. These thoughts become like a broken record that lulls us into complacency by making us believe that we can't change our life circumstances. "I could never make enough money doing what I love" or "I'm not attractive enough to find a great romantic partner" or "I'm not good enough" or "I'm not smart enough" or a myriad of other thoughts play over and over again in our minds. After years and years on repeat, we believe these thoughts are true.

Pause for a moment, take your finger off the repeat button, and ask yourself, "Are my self-limiting thoughts *really* true?" Do you have hard and fast evidence that you will *never* find the man or woman of your dreams? Are you really stuck at your job? What options haven't you considered? Keep an open mind while you ask yourself these questions. Treat it as a brainstorming exercise, where no idea is too far-fetched or wrong.

Maybe you can't afford to leave your job right now, but you could always sign up to receive job postings from Monster.com to keep you in the loop about new opportunities. Or maybe you're having trouble finding a romantic partner because you feel insecure about your body. Going for a bike ride a few times a week could give you the boost of confidence that you need to get out there and meet someone special.

To get off antidepressants for good, you need to stop seeing yourself as a victim of your life, and begin realizing that you are in control. Feel empowered by knowing that you are in control of your life – not the other way around. Even when bad things happen to us, we *always* have a choice about how we *react* to the situation. The classic example that Marci Shimoff uses in her book "*Happy for*

No Reason" is that of Victor Frankl, the author of *"Man's Search for Meaning."*

Victor Frankl was 37 years old when he, his wife, and his parents were sent to a concentration camp during World War II. In the camp, Victor experienced some of the worst hardships imaginable. He lost most of his loved ones (his wife and parents were murdered), and he had to give up all his material possessions. In *"Man's Search for Meaning,"* Victor wrote:

> *"We who lived in concentration camps can remember the men who walked through the huts comforting others, giving away their last piece of bread. They may have been few in number, but they offer sufficient proof that everything can be taken from a man but one thing: the last of human freedoms – to choose one's attitude in any given set of circumstances, to choose one's own way."*

You *always* have a choice about how you react to the things that happen to you. *No one* can take that away from you. You can choose to complain, be miserable, and feel defeated, or you can choose to grow and learn from your experiences. In *"Happy for No Reason"* Marci Shimoff calls it "looking for the lesson and the gift." There is always a lesson or gift that we can take from everything that happens to us.

Making smart choices can eliminate your need for antidepressants by allowing you to create a life that you love. In the end, you are *fully responsible* for creating the life you want, and no little happy pill is going to do it for you.

In their book *"Co-Active Coaching: New Skills for Coaching People Toward Success in Work and Life,"* Laura Whitworth, Karen Kimsey-House, Henry Kimsey-House, and Phillip Sandahl present the "Wheel of Life" exercise as a tool to evaluate how satisfied you are in eight areas of your life. These eight areas include:

- Career
- Money
- Health
- Friends and Family
- Significant Other/Romance
- Personal Growth
- Fun and Recreation
- Physical Environment

The Wheel of Life exercise asks you to rate each of these areas on a scale from 1 (*not at all satisfied*) to 10 (*completely satisfied*) in terms of how you feel about that area of your life today.

In this chapter, we will go through each of these eight areas to give you an idea of the types of choices you might need to make to help you get off antidepressants.

Career

Rate your current level of satisfaction with your career on a scale of 1 (*not at all satisfied*) to 10 (*completely satisfied*). Do you enjoy your job? If money wasn't an option, what would you be doing every day? What career opportunities exist for you that you might not have explored? What is your dream?

You might think that you're being fluffy or unrealistic by answering these questions. But the truth is that these questions hold the key to what will make you truly happy. A sacred Hindu text called *The Bhagavad Gita* suggests that we all have a *Dharma*, which means truth, nature's way, or righteousness. Each person's individual *Dharma*, commonly called one's *Svadharma*, reflects their true path. This path often relates to our natural inclinations and abilities. We know when something like a job just feels right. We also usually know when we're on the wrong path, although sometimes we're afraid to admit this to ourselves.

Following your *Dharma* will give you a sense of fulfillment and peace. Not following your *Dharma* often results in frustration, anxiety, and health problems. Even taking one small step toward your *Dharma* can help. For example, if you love creating homemade greeting cards, but feel you could never make enough money making cards full-time, you could still devote a few hours every week to card-making. Maybe you could even ask around at local shops to see if they would be willing to sell your creations. It's far better to follow your own *Dharma* than to work at a job just because society or a well-intentioned parent make you feel like you have to. The *Bhagavad Gita* notes:

> *"It is better to do your own dharma even imperfectly, than someone else's dharma perfectly. Even better to die in your dharma than in another's, which brings great fear."*

As I mentioned in the story at the beginning of this chapter, I left a perfectly good job that paid my bills so that I could follow my true purpose and write this book. For almost 2 years I kept pushing my true purpose down because I was terrified of not having a stable paycheck. Eventually my health started to be affected. I was miserable, despite the fact that I had everything society said would make me happy.

For awhile, I felt stuck at my job because my husband was unemployed, and we needed my income. But even then, I knew I had a choice. I chose to save as much money as I possibly could, even if it was only fifty or a hundred dollars here and there. Eventually, I saved up enough to support myself for a few months while I started my new business. So I left. And while not having a stable paycheck was somewhat stressful, it was nothing compared to the anguish I felt by staying at a job that literally sucked the life out of me.

At first, I was hesitant to tell my friends and family about my decision to leave my job. I thought they would chastise me for giving up a perfectly good source of income. To my surprise, my loved ones were unbelievably supportive. There's something about following your passion that inspires others. The people who knew me best could easily see that I was choosing to follow the path that was right for me. Even my former co-workers were enthusiastic supporters of my dream. It isn't always the case that your loved ones will support your career decisions, but if you stand by your beliefs, these people will eventually come around. In her book *"This Time I Dance! Creating the Work You Love,"* Harvard lawyer Tama Kieves describes how she left a lucrative corporate position to follow her dream of being a writer. At first, Tama's family wasn't overly supportive, but they eventually came to support her as she started to realize her dreams.

We often stay at our jobs because of money. But time and time again I see examples of people who are able to make plenty of money doing what they love – even if "what they love" involves writing, art, or some other unconventional form of income. You might be thinking that these people have a horseshoe up you know where – but often the only difference between them and you is that they were willing to take a risk to follow their dream. Tama Kieves went from being a Harvard lawyer to waiting tables so that she could live her true purpose. In describing her experiences, Tama writes:

> *"Gradually, I no longer saw myself as stepping down from a superior life, but stepping ahead into a life of artistic dignity and determination...I didn't want to linger in the corporate world just to prop myself up while I dragged my soul down. I'd rather bring out onion rings."*

So while you might think that you have no other option than to put up with your job, I'm here to tell you this simply isn't true. You *always* have other options. It just takes courage and determination to pursue those options. You might not even need to quit your job – maybe you just need to build up the courage to talk to your boss about that promotion you deserve, or mention the fact that you would like to work on a different type of project. It's up to you – but you owe it to yourself to follow your *Dharma*.

Money

How satisfied are you, on a scale of 1 to 10, with your financial situation? What's your relationship with money like? Do you have any destructive financial patterns? What unrealistic expectations do you have about money? Are you afraid of having too little money, or too much?

We often chain ourselves to the idea that we need to make a certain amount of money to be successful, or that we need to have some arbitrary amount of money in the bank at all times to be safe. Meanwhile, we rack up credit card debt so that we can keep up with the Jones', all the while wondering why our mounting material possessions don't seem to keep us happy for very long.

If your financial situation causes you stress, it's time to take a good hard look at your spending habits and expectations. Aside from typical monthly expenses like rent and bills, what do you spend the most money on? Are you hoarding money out of fear? Are you denying yourself pleasurable experiences, like that vacation you've always wanted to take? If you're racking up debt like crazy, examine your spending patterns. Why do you feel the need to spend beyond your means? Are you buying yourself things to soothe some part of you that's hurting from an unsatisfying job or relationship?

In my life, I've tended to take a fear-based approach to money. I was always afraid of not having enough, as if some sort of apocalypse was going to happen in which God would come down from the sky and ask me to pay Him a particular dollar amount to get into heaven. After quitting my job, I recognized my attachment to money, and decided to trust that I would always have enough to meet my needs. When I took a good hard look at my life, I realized that somehow the universe had always provided me with enough money. My family didn't have a lot of money when I was growing up, but somehow we made it through. I had to pay for my university education myself, but I always managed to find loans or scholarships to help me out. Even when money was really tight, I would often get an unexpected check from the government or a relative.

After quitting my job, I found it quite easy to reduce my expenses. I no longer felt the need to reward myself with an expensive dinner or a shopping spree after a crappy week at work. I soon realized that I had been spending a lot of my money on things that would make me feel better about the parts of my life I was unsatisfied with.

If you're constantly afraid that you won't have enough money, you will rob yourself of the opportunity to truly enjoy your life. So go on a vacation. Quit your job if it's killing you. You only have this life. That's it. Are you going to enjoy it, or spend all your time in fear?

Health

On a scale from 1 to 10, how satisfied are you with your physical health? What would being healthy feel or look like to you? Where are you holding back from living a healthy life? Are you avoiding your doctor and dentist appointments? What steps do you need to take to live a healthier lifestyle, even if you have a chronic health condition?

As I've mentioned in previous chapters, our physical bodies and our minds are intimately connected. If you don't take proper care of your body, your mind will suffer. Laying on the couch all day eating chips is definitely *not* going to help you feel less depressed. Similarly, exercising too much and obsessing over your body isn't going to help you feel less anxious. Being "healthy" isn't just about exercising all the time and following a crazy diet. You need to find a balance between physical activity and relaxation that works for you.

One healthy practice that can help you reduce anxiety is to eliminate caffeine from your diet. If you're a coffee lover, the previous sentence probably sent a wave of anxiety through your body! But a surprising number of people who suffer from anxiety fail to see the connection between caffeine and their symptoms. They drink coffee all day, then have trouble sleeping, then drink more coffee the next morning to combat their exhaustion. Often, these people have been drinking coffee for so many years that they don't attribute their feelings of anxiety to the caffeine. Instead, they think they're just chronically anxious. When they cut down their caffeine intake, they're amazed to realize that they aren't inherently anxious at all! If you suffer from anxiety, try cutting back on the caffeine and go for decaf instead. After the caffeine withdrawals fade, I guarantee you will feel less anxious.

Many experts also suggest cutting sugar out of your diet as a technique to deal with depression and anxiety.

This isn't something I've tried yet (I love chocolate too much!), but I've read quite a bit about how sugar wreaks havoc on our brain. Similar to caffeine, sugar props you up, gives you energy, and then sends you crashing down (usually at 3pm after lunch!). Try opting for sugar-free foods instead, and pay attention to how this effects your depression or anxiety.

The Ayurvedic principles discussed in Chapter 1 also suggest many dietary techniques to balance your mood. For example, if you tend to feel lethargic and slow, it might be best to avoid heavy, warm foods and opt for a salad instead. If, on the other hand, you have trouble slowing down, try calming your body with warm hearty soups and stews.

I'm not here to tell you exactly how much you should weigh, how much you should exercise, or what you should eat. Your body is inherently intelligent and often knows what's best. Pay attention to your body. Are you tired all the time? Maybe you need more sleep. Or maybe you need to introduce exercise into your life to give you more energy. Do your neck and shoulders ache? Maybe you need to adjust your desk at work or spend less time at the computer.

Use the advice of experts like doctors and naturopaths to help your body return to its naturally balanced state. Treat yourself to things like massages, facials, and pedicures. Dye your hair or get a new haircut if you need a boost. Start going to the gym or walk briskly for a half hour every night if you'd like to lose a few pounds. I'm not trying to suggest that physical appearances are of the utmost importance, but sometimes treating yourself to a little physical care can give you the energy and confidence you need to get off antidepressants.

As Cheryl Richardson suggests in her book *"The Art of Extreme Self-Care,"* it's important to make sure you're comfortable with the professionals who provide you with healthcare. If your doctor is rude, try to find a new one. If you're scared of the dentist, ask someone to come along with you for support.

And please don't let money be an issue when it comes to your health. It's often said that without your health, you have nothing. So take care of yourself! If you don't have insurance, see if you can trade services for care. For example, if you're a professional speaker, you could give a free lunch and learn at a spa in return for a pedicure. Many cities in the U.S. also have free medical clinics, or clinics that offer services on a sliding scale basis. Take care of your physical body, and your mental health will follow.

Friends and Family

How satisfied are you, on a scale of 1 to 10, with your relationships with friends and family? Do your friends and family support you or do they drag you down? Do you wish you had more friends? Where are you not being yourself with friends and family? Are you putting up with the behavior of a family member because you don't see how things could be any different? Are unhealthy patterns from your childhood resurfacing in your relationships with your friends?

Friends and family play an important role in our lives. As I've mentioned before, social support is extremely beneficial as a buffer against stress. Sometimes, however, we remain in unhealthy relationships with our friends and family – relationships that drain our energy and trap us in patterns that keep us on antidepressants. It's commonly said that we choose our friends, but we can't choose our family. And while this is largely true, it doesn't mean that we have to put up with family members who mistreat us.

You might notice that you tend to revert to childhood forms of anxiety when you speak to your father, or you get down in the dumps whenever you speak to your best friend who is a constant complainer. To get off antidepressants, you need to surround yourself with people who leave you feeling energized, upbeat, and full of potential. This doesn't mean you have to disown your family members or friends. What it does mean, however, is that you might have to make the choice to speak to your family less often, or avoid speaking to them about certain topics. Or you might need to have a frank conversation with your best friend about her tendency to complain.

While these sorts of decisions and conversations might not be easy, they are crucial to keeping you on the path toward antidepressant freedom. I love Cheryl Richardson's concept of *Extreme Self-Care* because she emphasizes the need for us to put ourselves first. Many people balk at this idea, thinking that they're being selfish by making themselves a priority. We often feel that we don't deserve to care for ourselves, and that we should put others first instead. Cheryl highlights the fact that if we don't care for ourselves, we limit our ability to effectively care for others. A good metaphor here is the idea of putting on your own oxygen mask in a plane crash before you try to fasten someone else's mask. If you don't give yourself enough air first, you'll be useless.

If a family member or friend is sucking your energy, you owe it to yourself to do something about it. Talk to the person, and if that doesn't work, you might need to end the relationship. Your health, time, and energy are too valuable to be taken away by others. Dealing with your toxic relationships can go a long way toward reducing your need for antidepressant medication.

Significant Other/Romance

I collapse onto my pillow as a heartfelt sob lurches up from my throat. My boyfriend and I have had yet another fight. He wants to be able to date other women at the same time as he dates me. We've been together for a couple of years, and on the one hand, I find his desire for an open relationship totally unacceptable. On the other hand, I'm so afraid of us breaking up that I figure I'm just going to have to give him what he wants.

During the fight, I tried to explain myself, telling him that I loved him and that I only wanted to be with him. He agreed that he loved me too, but that he also wanted to keep his options open. He had just moved away to university, and there were lots of girls in his dorm who seemed like good prospects. With his usual charisma, he refused to back down and persuaded me that his way was the right way.

I hung up the phone and sobbed for the next hour. I felt completely helpless. Why didn't he love me? Why couldn't I make him love me? Maybe if I was prettier, or taller, or more outgoing – maybe then he would finally commit. Exhausted from crying, I popped my daily dose of Paxil and hoped I would feel better in the morning.

~   ~   ~

Whether you're currently in a romantic relationship or not, rate your level of satisfaction with your romantic life on a scale from 1 to 10. Does your partner value you for who you truly are? Where are you settling in your relationship? What are your relationship patterns or habits? Would you like to have more, or less, romance in your life?

Even the best relationships get into funks sometimes. You might love your partner to death but feel you need a little more excitement. Or your partner might be doing something that really gets on your nerves that you've never brought up. Regardless of your current situation, it's important to assess what you love, and what's missing, from your romantic life.

If you need more excitement, you don't need to do anything drastic. Adding some zest to your relationship could be as simple as planning a day trip to a new town or joining a club together instead of plopping in front of the TV every night without speaking.

In fact, studies have shown that trying something new with your partner is linked to increases in relationship satisfaction. In one study, couples were tied together at the wrists and ankles and asked to crawl across a gymnasium while they pushed a foam cylinder with their heads – a task that was meant to be exciting and stimulating. These couples were compared to couples who were asked to sit still and slowly pass a ball back and forth to each other – a task that was meant to be relatively boring. Both groups of couples completed questionnaires assessing their relationship satisfaction before and after completing these tasks. The results showed that the couples who did the "exciting" task showed greater increases in their relationship satisfaction from before to after the task than couples who did the boring task. If something as simple as pushing a foam cylinder with your head can improve your relationship quality, then surely there's hope for even the most boring relationships!

If there's one thing I learned from studying romantic relationships while doing my Ph.D. in psychology, it's that it takes hard work to maintain your relationship satisfaction over time. At the core of this hard work are good communication skills. If there's something bothering you about your partner, you need to talk about it. Sweeping it under the rug is just going to make it fester.

When communicating with your partner, try not to be defensive. Even if you don't agree with what your partner is saying, you can still appreciate why they're feeling upset or hurt. Validate your partner's feelings by telling them that you understand their point of view. Then, if you would like, explain your point of view. When providing this explanation, use "I" language. For example, instead of saying "You never help me out around the house," try, "It makes me feel unappreciated when you don't help me out around the house."

Most of all, when you're discussing an area of conflict with your partner, try to keep the discussion as positive as possible. Studies have shown that couples who stay together over time tend to engage in 5 positive behaviors for every 1 negative behavior when they discuss an area of conflict with their partner. Couples who divorce, on the other hand, tend to show 0.8 positive behaviors for every 1 negative behavior during conflict discussions. In other words, couples who stay together don't *avoid* negativity – but they *buffer* negativity with lots of positivity.

Dr. John Gottman, a leading researcher on marriage and relationships, has actually developed methods that can predict, with over 90% accuracy, which couples will divorce – based simply on observing a 15-minute conflict discussion between the couple. Couples who end up divorcing tend to show very specific interaction patterns when they discuss an area of conflict. Dr. Gottman calls these interaction patterns "The Four Horsemen of the Marriage Apocalypse." These are four communication styles that you should try to avoid when discussing an area of conflict with your partner, and include:

- **Criticism**. Criticism involves expressing negative evaluations of your partner, highlighting their faults, and attacking their personality or character. For example, "You're so irresponsible for not taking out the garbage." Women are more likely to criticize than men.

- **Contempt**. Contempt involves being insulting toward your partner, and expressing superiority. This is often a sign of disrespect for your partner. For example, putting your partner down, rolling your eyes, or sneering.

- **Defensiveness**. Being defensive involves responding to a perceived attack by your partner with obstructive communication that escalates the conflict. For example, denying responsibility, making excuses, or meeting one complaint with another.

- **Stonewalling.** Stonewalling involves refusing to listen to your partner and withdrawing from the interaction. For example, refusing to communicate or being unresponsive. Men tend to stonewall more than women.

All couples show these behaviors every once in awhile. But try to avoid using the Four Horsemen as your primary way of communicating with your partner when you discuss an area of conflict. Dr. Gottman's research spans 35 years and is quite vast – those who are interested in reading more about his work should visit www.gottman.com.

Another important thought to consider about your romantic relationship is whether you're settling. Sometimes it's easier for us to stay with a partner who we're not really meant to be with, simply because we're afraid of being alone. Don't let fear motivate you to stay in an unsatisfying relationship. Sure, breaking up might be hard, but it will also give you the time and space to learn more about yourself and about what you really want to get out of your relationships. And who knows, the perfect partner could be right around the corner.

As the story at the beginning of this section suggests, I was involved in a relationship for 6 years that was quite dysfunctional. We were high school sweethearts, and spent most of our early 20s together. He was smart, athletic, good looking, and we had a lot in common. But he was also very manipulative, often convincing me to do things or to get into situations that I was uncomfortable with. As I described in the story above, he wanted us to have an open relationship. He often kept me a secret from his friends in the hope of dating other women while he was also dating me.

I expressed my dissatisfaction with his behavior, but he was so charismatic and convincing that he was always able to persuade me that we were meant to be together. I tried to loosen his grip on me by breaking up with him several times, but I always went back. I was studying psychology at the time in a largely female program, and I wasn't into meeting new people at bars. I was certain that I would never meet anyone else, and that he and I had enough in common to make things work.

I originally went on antidepressants partly because of the anxiety and sadness that I was experiencing about this relationship. Throughout the relationship, I tried several times to get off antidepressants, but always ended up back on them. My partner made me feel insecure, nervous, and unworthy of commitment. When I moved away to attend graduate school, I finally got up the courage to end the relationship once and for all. This was not an easy task. I had just moved to a new city where I didn't know anyone, and I was about to start my Masters degree in a very competitive program. But I finally decided to choose myself over my dysfunctional relationship.

The following year wasn't easy. I went in and out of several messy relationships as I tried to regain my self-esteem. Eventually I decided to join an online dating website. When I first joined the site, I kept it a secret from many of my friends and family. I was embarrassed that I had to resort to online dating to meet someone, and I thought this meant I was desperate. I mean really – I was smart, I was reasonably attractive – why couldn't I just meet someone the "normal" way?

This is a perfect example of the type of limited thinking that can chain us to our old patterns and habits, because if I hadn't gotten up the courage to do something a little different by trying online dating, I never would have met my husband.

Today I'm happily married because I was brave enough to get out of a dysfunctional relationship and try online dating. When my ex found out that I was getting involved in a serious relationship, he went through a valiant effort to win back my attention. He blogged about me, he drove over an hour to show up unexpectedly at my office, and he even sent me a DVD recording of himself singing songs that professed his love. My new boyfriend, who is now my husband, recognized that my ex's behavior was irrational and even bordered on stalking. So my husband gave me a choice – either cut off all communication with my ex, or our budding relationship would end.

On the surface, this ultimatum may seem overprotective or controlling, and at first I even interpreted it that way. I had been best friends with my ex since high school, and our friendship was important to me. But my husband saw how the relationship affected me. He could see through my ex's manipulative tactics, and he was scared that someday my ex's controlling behavior might get out of hand.

So I cut off all ties with my ex, and we haven't spoken since. Again, this was not an easy decision to make. At his core, I believe my ex is a good person – he just had his own issues that he needed to deal with. But the truth of the matter was that if I wanted my new relationship to work, I couldn't maintain a friendship with my ex. If I was going to increase my self-confidence and get off antidepressants, I needed to cut my ex out of my life for good.

Luckily, my husband helped me make the right decision. I knew I deserved better, and while cutting my ex out of my life wasn't easy, it led me to where I am today. I could have taken the easy route, married my high school sweetheart – and ended up miserable. If I had taken that path, I would probably still be on antidepressants today because of the way my old relationship made me feel.

Fortunately, I had the courage to find someone who treats me like gold. Do you?

No matter how stuck you feel in your relationship, or how long it's been since you've dated someone, there are options out there for you to meet new people. Try joining a dating website like www.lavalife.com or www.eharmony.com. Or go out to a singles night or a speed dating event in your city. It's up to you to create the relationship of your dreams – and it is possible.

Personal Growth

On a scale of 1 to 10, how satisfied are you with your personal growth? Do you feel you devote enough time to self-development? Do you ever do things just for you, not for anyone else? What does the term "personal growth" mean to you? What would your life look like if you devoted 1 day per month to self-development?

On the surface, the term "personal growth" might seem a little fluffy or new age. However, personal growth doesn't have to mean anything spiritual or airy fairy. Instead, personal growth represents the things that you do to enhance your self-concept – things that you enjoy, that make you feel good, and that contribute to your growth as a person.

For example, to enhance your personal growth, you might decide to take an evening course at a continuing education center in your city. Or you might choose to spend at least two hours per week learning about local perennials and tending to your garden. Or you might have a passion for cars, and decide to learn about how to refurbish old Hondas in your spare time.

As adults, we often believe that our time for learning is over. Sure, we learn from life experiences, but all too often we assume that it doesn't make sense for us to try something new. We think we're too old, or that we don't have enough time. But it's important to *make* the time for our own self-development. You're never too old to try something new. When my stepfather went blind, he decided to learn how to play the drums, and ended up being part of several bands around town. He also took up weight-lifting and made quite a name for himself locally as a blind bodybuilder. If someone can get shot in the face, lose their sight, and go on to learn completely new hobbies, certainly you can pick up the yellow pages and join a local club.

Stop putting others ahead of yourself and start pursuing things that make you feel fulfilled and joyful. As you do, you'll eliminate the need for an antidepressant to make you happy.

Fun and Recreation

It's Friday, and I'm feeling stressed because I didn't accomplish as much at work this week as I think I should have. As I drive home from the office, my mind races with all the tasks that I still need to do. Maybe I should just work through the evening so that I can get everything done. But I'm supposed to go to a cottage for the weekend to hang out at the beach with friends. "How can I possibly take time off this weekend, when I have so much to do?" I think as I pull into my driveway. My husband greets me at the door, chipper and ready for the weekend. His smile slowly fades as I tell him that I've decided to stay home this weekend to get work done. "But you've been working so hard this week," he implores, "a weekend at the beach will do you some good!" Reluctantly, I decide to leave the work at home and head to the cottage.

It's July. The sky is perfectly blue, and the sun is setting brightly over the farmer's fields as we drive out of the city. I take a deep breath of fresh air. After only a half hour in the car, I realize that my husband was right. I'm already feeling my anxiety melt away. We end up having a great time at the beach. After the weekend is over, I'm refreshed and ready to tackle anything that comes my way on Monday morning.

~   ~   ~

On a scale of 1 to 10, how satisfied are you with the amount of fun in your life? Do you take the time to have fun on a regular basis? What do you do purely for fun – without any sense of obligation? What steps could you take to bring more fun into your life?

Maybe you think you don't have enough time for fun. Between work and family obligations, it might feel like fun is an elusive concept, only to be enjoyed by the rich and famous. But a life without fun is pretty dreary. Cutting fun out of your life makes you feel lethargic and low – which keeps you attached to antidepressants.

There must be something – anything – that you enjoy doing, just for the sake of doing it. Maybe you like going for walks, or collecting stamps, or bird watching. Whatever it is – make time for it. There's almost always something you can say no to in your life in order to say yes to fun. When it comes to balancing work with play, Cheryl Richardson, author of *"The Art of Extreme Self-Care,"* recommends making two lists: an absolute no list and an absolute yes list.

- **The Absolute Yes List**. Reflect on your top priorities – for example your health, children, or volunteer work. Narrow these priorities down to your top seven, and make a commitment to yourself to devote your time and energy first and foremost to these things. When making a decision about how to spend your time – ask yourself, "Does this reflect a priority on my absolute yes list?" For example, if your boss asks you to work on the weekend, see if this is in line with your top priorities. If it's not an absolute yes, then it's a no.

- **The Absolute No List**. Creating an absolute no list involves reflecting on the things that sap your time and energy. For example, you might hate gardening but feel pressure to maintain your lawn, or you might despise doing the laundry. Or maybe you're tired of being available for work at all hours on your Blackberry. To make your absolute no list, start with the sentence "I no longer..." and fill in the blanks with as many items as you wish. To go along with the examples above, you might say

"I no longer garden. Instead, I pay someone to do my landscaping," or "I no longer do the laundry. Instead, I teach my husband how to do it," or "I no longer respond to work emails after 6pm on my Blackberry."

Your absolute yes and no lists help you make time for fun by clarifying what's important to you, as well as what you will no longer tolerate. It's commonly said that when we're on our deathbed, we seldom look back and wish we'd spent more time at the office or in front of the TV. Say yes to fun by choosing to engage in activities that lift your spirits and make you feel good – even if this means saying no to something else.

We often feel that we have to control everything around us, which makes us scared to delegate tasks to others. Try handing off a few tasks. I guarantee the world will not end. Eventually you'll realize that someone else can tend your garden just as well as you can, or that your husband is an intelligent human being who is perfectly capable of doing the laundry himself without flooding the house or turning everything pink. By filling your life with more of what you want, and less of what you don't want, it becomes much easier to release your need for antidepressants.

Physical Environment

How satisfied are you, on a scale from 1 to 10, with the environments that you spend most of your time in? What do you like or not like about your house or apartment? What do you enjoy or not enjoy about your office? What would the ideal house, apartment, or workplace look like for you? What steps can you take to bring your current physical environment closer to your ideal?

We often pay very little attention to our physical surroundings. But the characteristics of the places where we spend our time can have a profound effect on our sense of well-being. Think about how you feel when you walk into a favorite room in your house, or when you enter a yoga studio or a gym. In these places, you most likely experience a sense of calm and peace. Think about how you feel when you see a nice bouquet of flowers on a table. Almost immediately you get a sense of beauty and energy. Now think of an environment that you don't enjoy – perhaps your office at work or a room in your house that's under renovations. When you enter these spaces, you most likely feel anxious and uptight.

To feel well, it's important for us to nurture our minds by surrounding ourselves with things that make us feel good. If your home or office is cluttered, try practicing the yogic principle of *sauca*, or purity, by eliminating the things you don't need. You'll be amazed at how inspired and energetic you'll feel when you get rid of your clutter. If you sit in a cubicle at work that's rather dismal, try putting up some pictures of friends and family, or buy some flowers for your desk. If your house feels cold and dark in the winter, invest in some cozy slippers and a couple of warmly-lit lamps to spruce things up.

In *"The Art of Extreme Self-Care,"* Cheryl Richardson suggests a four step process to create what she calls a "soul-loving space:"

- **Examine**. Reflect on whether the spaces where you work and live nurture your soul or rob you of energy.
- **Evaluate**. Figure out what you need to change in the energy-sapping environments to create a more inspiring space.
- **Eliminate**. Get rid of things you don't need, by recycling, giving them to friends and family, or donating them to charity.
- **Enhance**. Improve your new space by adding elements to it that inspire you and represent who you really are.

Following these four steps might be challenging at first, especially the act of giving things away! But by surrounding yourself with a physical environment that expresses your unique tastes and values, you'll create a sense of inner peace and happiness that will lessen your need for antidepressants.

Finding Balance

Picture a pie with each of the eight areas of your life described above as one slice: career, money, health, friends and family, significant other/romance, personal growth, fun and recreation, and physical environment. The size of each slice corresponds to how satisfied you rated yourself, on a scale of 1 to 10, with each area. Step back and look at how your pie is sliced. Are the pieces of relatively equal size? Are some pieces huge while other pieces are just slivers? Why are some pieces bigger or smaller than others? Are there any pieces that you would like to make bigger or smaller?

Making changes in multiple areas of your life all at once can be overwhelming. You don't need to "fix" everything all at the same time. In fact, if you try to take on too much, you can end up overwhelmed and easily sink back into your old habits. Start by working on one area that represents a particularly unsatisfying piece of your pie. Don't pressure yourself to suddenly create a perfect life – start small and eventually you'll get there.

Starting small is especially important as you're getting off antidepressants. In most cases, it's best to make any major life changes while you're still on the medication, and then begin tapering off once your life has calmed down. While it's true that this means it might take longer to get off the drugs, the benefits are well worth it. Over time, you'll have created a life for yourself that makes it *much* easier for you to get off antidepressants, and facilitates your ability to stay off the drugs over the long term.

Creating a balanced and fulfilling life is a continuous journey that never really ends. There's almost always something you could improve about your circumstances with a little effort. As an example, last month I decided that for the time being, I'm no longer going to take care of my garden. For years I've felt stressed about my garden looking nice – to the point where it just wasn't fun to garden anymore. I don't have the money right now to pay someone to pull weeds for me, so I'm just letting my garden grow. The odd time I'll go out and spend a few minutes snipping some branches or dead-heading a couple of flowers, but that's it. My garden looks like a jungle – but I've never felt better about it. I released the attachment I had to my garden looking like something out of a magazine, and I'm just allowing it to be beautiful and natural as it is.

As another example, when I landed a job after finishing my Ph.D., one of the first things I did was hire someone to clean my house on a regular basis. I didn't do this because I'm lazy or because I'm incapable of tidying up. I did it because I wanted to spend less time cleaning, and more time doing the things I love. When I quit my job to write this book, I had no stable form of income. I cut many of my expenses, but I kept my cleaning lady. This cost me precious money, but it was money that I was willing to spend so that I had time to do things that nourished my soul like yoga, reading, and walking in nature.

When we say yes or no to one thing in life, we're almost always saying yes or no to something else. For example, by saying no to my garden this year, I'm saying yes to weeds, and also saying yes to the possibility that my friends or neighbors might think my garden is ugly. By saying yes to my cleaning lady, I'm saying no to housework, and also saying yes to freeing up my time to do things I enjoy. If you say no to your boss's request for you to work on the weekend, you might be saying yes to more time with your family, but also saying no to a pay increase.

When you make choices, always be aware of everything you're saying yes and no to. As another example, when I was finishing my Ph.D., I said no to several opportunities that came my way, such as the chance to teach a course and an opportunity to review several manuscripts in a prestigious journal. I made this choice because I wanted to finish my thesis on time. Instead of teaching the course to make money, I took out a student loan. By not teaching the course and not reviewing those manuscripts, I went into a bit of debt and missed out on a possibility to increase my presence in my field of research. But I also managed to stay sane, finish my thesis on time, and spend some quality time with my friends and family.

As yet another example, I very seldom worked evenings or weekends at my job, even though many of my colleagues did so regularly. By saying no to weekend work, it's possible that I hurt my chances of earning extra commission or getting a faster promotion. My coworkers might have also thought I was somewhat antisocial when I chose to do my work instead of spending time chatting with them at the water cooler. But these were sacrifices I was willing to make so that I could spend time outside of work doing things I enjoyed.

In her book *"The Art of Extreme Self-Care,"* Cheryl Richardson has an excellent chapter called "Let Me Disappoint You." The chapter talks about how most of us hate to disappoint others, but that disappointing others is often an inevitable consequence of caring for ourselves. For example, your spouse or children might be disappointed when you decide to take a Sunday just for yourself, or your boss might be disappointed when you turn down the opportunity to work on a new project. But to go back to the analogy of the oxygen mask on the airplane – you need to take care of yourself before you can effectively care for others.

I urge you to choose yourself. Regardless of your specific situation, you *always* have a choice. You can choose to put up with the parts of your life that drain your energy, or you can harness the courage to make a change. When you're 95 years old, looking back on your life, what will you want to say about it?

It's your life. And it's your call.

List of Resources

- *"Happy for No Reason: 7 Steps to Being Happy from the Inside Out"* by Marci Shimoff.
- *"Man's Search for Meaning"* by Victor Frankl.
- *"Co-Active Coaching: New Skills for Coaching People Toward Success in Work and Life"* by Laura Whitworth, Karen Kimsey-House, Henry Kimsey-House, and Phillip Sandahl.
- *"The Living Gita: The Complete Bhagavad Gita"* with commentary by Sri Swami Satchidananda.
- *"This Time I Dance! Creating the Work You Love"* by Tama Kieves.
- *"The Art of Extreme Self-Care"* by Cheryl Richardson.
- Dr. John Gottman's relationship research: www.gottman.com.
- Dating websites: www.lavalife.com or www.eharmony.com.

Chapter 5
Step 5 – Blend Thoroughly and Repeat As Necessary

I remember fat noodles. My husband had promised to make dinner, but he seemed a bit out of sorts and had overcooked the pasta. The noodles had turned into waterlogged sponges and were sticking to the bottom of the pot. I arrived home late after proctoring an exam on campus. I'd been off antidepressants for 3 years, and I was in the process of finishing my Ph.D.

"What's wrong?" I asked.

"Nothing, I'm just busy." He replied as he plopped a mound of congealed noodles onto my plate.

We ate mostly in silence, and I could tell he was preoccupied.

After dinner he finally admitted that he had something to tell me. He started off with a few sentences that were supposed to soften the main message. However, I only remember two words: "Paul died."

At this point my memory becomes fragmented, like someone took a reel of film from an old movie and chopped pieces out of it. I see a tear rolling down my husband's right cheek, then I blink for what seems like a moment and I find myself in the bathroom crying. I blink again and I'm staring at my bedroom ceiling trying to sleep. I blink again and I'm on campus the next morning with puffy eyes, putting something in a colleague's mailbox because I know I'll be away for a few days.

The next time I open my eyes I'm in the car on the way to my home town. I blink, then I'm in a hotel room getting ready to see my mother. My memories continue like this, as shards of light between periods of darkness. At times, I sense things with perfect clarity and detail: the corner of my cousin's mouth as she greets me at the funeral. The loud wind ripping through the trees as I try to sleep. The smell of stale cigarettes as I walk into my childhood home. My father's blue sweater slung over his favorite chair. A pink Oxycontin pill contrasting starkly against the grey pavement of the basement floor.

When people speak, it sounds like we're underwater. I can see their mouths moving, but their words fall flat, struggling to get through the murky liquid between us. Somehow I manage to smile at the right times, say the right things, and put one foot in front of the other.

The next time I open my eyes my mother and I are alone in the living room. The funeral reception is over, and everyone has left. I can hear the second-hand moving on the clock in the dining room. Everything is slow and empty, but there's a palpable fullness around us. Mounds of sandwiches sit piled on the kitchen table, reminding us of all the people who were supposed to show up but didn't. I blink, and then we're crying, holding each other. The moment is brief. The next time I open my eyes my husband and I are in the car, heading back to the city.

In retrospect, I know that hours and even days were passing between these memories. But they have been preserved in my mind as brief flashbulbs in time, separated by long shadows.

~   ~   ~

The world doesn't magically turn into a peaceful and loving place after you get off antidepressants. You will need to continually draw from the steps outlined in this book to help you stay off antidepressants for good.

The story above describes the very tragic and unexpected death of my stepfather Paul. I've mentioned Paul several times throughout this book, both as an example of someone with incredible perseverance in the face of adversity, as well as a person who added significant stress to my life.

Paul died after I'd been off antidepressants for 3 years. Two months earlier, my mother had left him. He'd become impossible to live with after he developed chronic pain and became addicted to Oxycontin. Paul had been shot in the face in his early 20s and lost his sight as a result. After this attempted murder, he cleaned up his life, joined AA, and hadn't touched a drop of alcohol in over 25 years. But his addictive personality stayed with him, and when his GP put him on Oxycontin for his chronic pain, he quickly became dependent on it.

After my mom left him, his behavior got worse. He started selling things in my childhood home to get money to buy Oxycontin illegally. He was extremely conflicted about his addiction, and even stopped going to AA meetings because he felt like a hypocrite. In the past, he'd often spoken at these meetings, and in local prisons, to inspire people to turn their lives around. In the end, he was angry and isolated, lashing out at everyone who loved him. For the last two months of his life he lived alone, even going so far as to remove all the light bulbs from the lamps in his house so that anyone who visited at night would have to endure the darkness like him.

He died alone, on his bedroom floor. He was 55 years old. And he was the only father I'd ever known.

Two weeks before his death, I was visiting my mom for Thanksgiving, so I drove by his house to pay him a visit. There was a "For Sale" sign on the front lawn, and the grass hadn't been cut in weeks. I drove around the block several times but I just couldn't bring myself to knock on the door. I was uncomfortable with everything about the situation – his addiction, his behavior, and the fact that I was experiencing a second father figure who had given up on his family. So I drove away.

I never saw him again.

He died when I was in the final year of finishing my Ph.D. thesis. At the time, I was also completing an intensive yoga teacher training certification program. This was a year that was already stressful enough on its own. Taken together, these events could have easily driven me back into the arms of antidepressants. But I managed to stay antidepressant-free throughout my stepfather's death, and went on to successfully complete my Ph.D. in psychology, become a certified yoga teacher, and land a well-paying job.

How did I do it? By continually applying and re-applying the steps outlined in this book.

To review, here is a brief summary of my five step antidepressant antidote program:

- **Step 1 – Get Help.** To get off antidepressants, you need to uncover and deal with the issues that got you on the medication in the first place. To do this, I strongly suggest you see a therapist. I also recommend you lean on your friends and family for support, while also working with your doctor. Finally, I suggest you make use of several forms of alternative medicine, such as naturopathy, Ayurveda, Reiki, and Thai massage.

- **Step 2 – Kick the Habit.** Going off antidepressants can cause both physical and psychiatric withdrawal symptoms, like crying spells, anxiety, nausea, dizziness, and electrical "zapping" sensations in your body. It's *extremely* important to taper off antidepressants slowly to reduce the likelihood that you will experience withdrawal effects. Work with your doctor to make sure you're ready to go off antidepressants, and use his or her expertise to find a tapering program that's right for you.

- **Step 3 – Let Go.** Anxiety often involves worrying about the future, while depression typically involves feeling sad about the past. Use techniques like meditation, yoga, and breathing exercises to bring your attention into the present moment. These practices were essential in helping me get off antidepressants. If yoga isn't your thing, try some other form of physical activity like karate or tai chi or an aerobics class.

- **Step 4 – Choose Wisely.** It's often easier for us to stick with the status quo of our current jobs, relationships, and patterns, than to make the sometimes tough choices that will move us toward antidepressant freedom. To feel happy and at peace without antidepressants, we have to make a conscious decision to get rid of the personal and professional shackles that chain us to the medication. Evaluate your life to see where you might need to make some changes.

- **Step 5 – Blend Thoroughly and Repeat as Necessary.** As I describe in more detail below, you will need to repeatedly sample from these five steps, in no particular order, throughout your journey. Even though I've been off antidepressants for 5 years, I still use many of the principles outlined in this book as part of my ongoing effort to manage my stress and mood. Combine these five steps in any way you like to create your own blueprint for antidepressant freedom.

How to Stay Antidepressant-Free Over the Long Haul

As I mentioned in the Introduction, the steps in this book don't necessarily appear in chronological order. Similar to the eight limbs of yoga, these five steps are better thought of as parts of a spiral. Over time, you will travel up and down the spiral, continuously sampling from and building on each component.

Even after you get off antidepressants, you will probably need to draw on the help provided by friends, family, and maybe even doctors and therapists as you go through the typical trials and tribulations of life (Step 1 – Get Help). You might even need to go back on antidepressants at some point and then try to get off them again later (Step 2 – Kick the Habit). You will need to engage in practices that help you let go of thoughts and patterns that burden you (Step 3 – Let Go), and you will need to make wise choices to keep you on your true path (Step 4 – Choose Wisely).

This is why I call Step 5 *"Blend Thoroughly and Repeat as Necessary."* Staying off antidepressants is a continuous journey that doesn't end simply because you've stopped taking your pills. Remember that in most cases, you ended up on the pills for a reason. Now whether or not that reason necessitated the use of medication is a whole other matter. Regardless, there was something going on for you at some point in your life that led to the use of antidepressants. At times throughout the rest of your life, these circumstances or issues might come back to haunt you. When they do, you need to be armed, ready, and resilient with the tactics and techniques outlined in this book.

These five steps represent a holistic way for you to approach personal healing. To get off antidepressants, you need to heal your *whole* being – body, mind, and spirit. Humans are complex, multifaceted beings, and it's overly simplistic to think that one magic bullet is going to cure all your problems. This is why I recommend using these five steps *in combination* with each other. When I was going off antidepressants, I was seeing a therapist, my doctor, and a naturopath. I was also doing yoga, meditating, getting Reiki treatments, going for Thai massages, and talking to my friends and family about what I was going through. These treatments and services took time and cost money, but the result was well worth it.

In the end, getting off antidepressants often comes down to personal responsibility. You are *fully responsible* for doing the best you can to create a life that will eliminate your need for antidepressants. As I've mentioned many times throughout this book, there are some cases in which antidepressants are absolutely necessary. In most other cases, however, people can often eliminate their need for antidepressants by taking personal responsibility for their health and well-being.

I agree with Ayurvedic practitioners who emphasize that our body knows how to heal itself. Take the example of cutting your finger. Your body immediately mobilizes to heal the wound and close it over. Why should we think of our mental healing any differently? You intuitively know how to heal your mental wounds and get off antidepressants. You know what you need to do to bring more happiness and relaxation into your life. Listen to that small, still voice inside of you that's asking you to follow your true path. The five steps in this book are meant to help you listen to the only guru you will ever need – yourself. The choices you need to make might not be easy, but you know what they are. And you owe it to yourself to make them.

I wish I could use a magic wand to send all your troubles away with a confident "poof!" Unfortunately, no such wand exists, not even in the form of modern medicine. Staying off antidepressants over the long haul takes hard work, courage, and determination. It takes the type of person who is willing to stand up for themselves and make their health and well-being their number one priority. You will need to be true to yourself and make choices that allow you to live an authentic life – a life of purpose, fulfillment, and balance – even if this means occasionally disappointing others.

As I mentioned in the Introduction, this is not a journey for the faint of heart. But trust me, your hard work and determination will not be in vain.

If At First You Don't Succeed,
Try and Try Again

Throughout this book I've frequently mentioned that I tried several times to get off antidepressants before I was finally able to shake the drugs for good. If you experience a setback, simply pick yourself up, dust yourself off, and start again. The steps in this book provide you with a toolkit that you can draw on at any time to help you out along the way.

Right now just might not be the right time for you to get off antidepressants. Maybe you have too many changes or life stressors going on, or perhaps you haven't fully worked through your issues with a qualified professional. During most of my unsuccessful attempts to get off antidepressants, I was usually experiencing some sort of life stressor. For example, at one point I was stuck in the dysfunctional relationship that I described in the last chapter. Another time I had just gotten out of that dysfunctional relationship. And yet another time I was just about to finish my Masters thesis. But I kept trying.

Every time I went back on antidepressants, I always reminded myself that I could try again in the future. I was determined to try as many times as it took to eventually get off the drugs. No one can chain you to antidepressants for the rest of your life except yourself. Obviously, if you have a severe psychiatric condition that robs you of your ability to function without antidepressants, then you might need to be on medication for a long time. But I agree with Joseph Glenmullen, M.D., author of "*Prozac Backlash*," that 75% of the people who are currently taking antidepressants can significantly reduce their dose or stop taking antidepressants completely (with the help of their doctor and other lifestyle changes).

It wasn't until I was in a relatively calm, secure period in my life that I was able to get off antidepressants for good. I was in a healthy, stable relationship. I was completing the second year of my Ph.D., which meant I had finished my comprehensive exams as well as most of my coursework, and I was practicing yoga regularly. I had been in therapy for 6 years, and I had processed a lot of my issues. It was a long journey, but it was well worth it.

Take your time and be gentle with yourself when getting off antidepressants. Your patience will be rewarded in the end with antidepressant freedom. Even if it takes you years to finally taper off the medication, that's ok. As Lao-tzu, author of the *Tao Te Ching* professed, "The journey of a thousand miles begins with a single step." Each step you take toward antidepressant freedom, no matter how small, is helping you attain your goal.

My Ongoing Journey

Since getting off antidepressants 5 years ago, my life has been an incredible journey of learning and self-exploration. I'm so relieved to be rid of the antidepressant side effects that plagued me for many years. And I'm amazed at the benefits that practices like yoga, meditation, breathwork, therapy, naturopathy, Ayurveda, Reiki, Thai Massage, and making smart choices have had on my anxiety and sadness.

As I mentioned at the beginning of this chapter, my antidepressant-free life hasn't been a walk in the park. Here are some of the things I've been through since going off antidepressants:

- My mother and stepfather separated.
- My stepfather died suddenly and tragically.
- I finished my Ph.D.

- I completed a 200-hour yoga teacher training course.
- I started a new job that was completely out of my field.
- I got married (ugh, wedding planning!).
- I bought a new house.
- I quit my well-paying job, with no new source of income, so that I could write this book.

These events have caused me to experience a world of emotions, from excruciating sadness to heart-lifting bliss. I've come to realize that these emotions are a *normal* part of life. I wasn't depressed when I crumpled onto the floor in tears after my stepfather died, and I wasn't manic or bipolar when I couldn't sleep from the excitement of having finished my Ph.D. I now strive to see life as an adventure – a journey that has ups and downs that I'm perfectly capable of handling without medication.

You might be saying to yourself, "She's so motivated and determined – I could never do what she's done" or "My life has been way worse than hers – I need antidepressants to help me deal with my problems." I'm here to tell you that in all likelihood, you're wrong. You *can* get off antidepressants. The only difference between you and me is that I stopped listening to the self-limiting thoughts that were telling me I was a chronically anxious person who would need to take antidepressants for the rest of my life.

I truly believe that I will never need to take antidepressants again. Now of course, anything can happen, and if I ever became so anxious or sad that I couldn't function, I would *maybe* need to consider medication. But I am 99.99% sure this will never happen. Why? Because I now have the tools, resources, and resiliency to keep me off antidepressants over the long haul.

I still have days when I feel anxious or sad, but now I see these emotions as being a natural part of life. If I filled out some sort of anxiety questionnaire today, I would probably still be classified as "high strung" or "Type A." But this doesn't mean that I need medication. When I feel anxious, it means that I need to get myself onto my yoga mat, or talk to a friend, or simply take a break. Everyone has bad days. Just because you have a bad day every once in awhile, it doesn't mean you need to be on antidepressants.

A couple of years ago, one of my aunts asked me an interesting question. We were sitting in her kitchen after a couple of glasses of wine. She looked me straight in the eyes, smiled, and asked, "How did you do it?"

"Do what?" I asked, slightly confused.

She clarified, "How did you create this life for yourself? I mean, no offence, but your childhood kind of sucked, your father abandoned you, hardly anyone in our family has ever been to university, but somehow you persevered and became so successful. How did you do it?"

I must admit that at the time I didn't know how to respond. I'd never really thought about it. Dumfounded, I rambled on about a few things, but I didn't really feel satisfied with my answer.

I now realize that this book is the answer to my aunt's question. This is how I did it.

These five steps don't only represent how I got off antidepressants. They also describe how I've managed to persevere in life even when things seemed difficult or hopeless. Deep down inside, I've always believed in myself and I know that even in my most insecure moments, I'm capable of making my life into whatever I want it to be. No person or life circumstance can *ever* take that away from me. And no one can take it away from you, either.

You *always* have a choice when it comes to living your best life.

What do you choose?

An Invitation

"Every creative contribution makes its way into
the world through the love of unseen hands."
—Tama Kieves

I would like to invite you to share this book with others. Recommend it to your friends, family, doctors, naturopaths, local bookstores – anyone who you think would benefit from the information I provide.

I quit my full-time job to write this book because I truly believe it has the potential to help many people. There are 118 million prescriptions written for antidepressants in the U.S. every year. If I could reach even a fraction of these people with this book, I would be doing my life's work. It is part of my life's true purpose to share the five steps in this book, and from this pure place in my heart I'm asking you to share my message by recommending this book to others.

Here are a few ways you can get involved:

- Visit my website at www.bethanybutzer.com to learn more about my life coaching services, workshops, and yoga classes.
- Follow me on Facebook by "Liking" my profile page at www.facebook.com/pages/London-ON/Bethany-Butzer-PhD-Mental-Health-Wellness-Advisor/117943314924607.
- Email me at bethany@bethanybutzer.com to sign up for my FREE monthly e-newsletter, which provides tips on enhancing your well-being.
- Invite me to present my *"Antidepressant Antidote: Five Steps to Get Off Antidepressants Safely and Effectively"* workshop at your wellness center, workplace, or anywhere else in your community where we can find the space.
- Contact me with any feedback you have about this book. I would love to hear your story of getting off antidepressants, and how my message helped you.
- Get in touch with me about any ideas you might have for us to collaborate – I love working with other wellness professionals to help people achieve their dreams.

I can't wait to spread my *"Antidepressant Antidote"* message around the world. Thank-you so much for supporting my efforts by purchasing this book. Feel free to get in touch with me any time – I would love to hear from you.

Warmly,

Bethany Butzer, Ph.D.
Mental Health & Wellness Advisor

bethany@bethanybutzer.com
www.bethanybutzer.com

With Thanks

You are holding this book in your hands not only because of my efforts. This book was made possible through the unwavering support of many people.

First, I would like to thank Hay House publishing for opening Balboa Press in the same week that I decided to quit my job to write this book (the universe works in mysterious ways!). I am continually inspired by the high quality, soulful books and conferences that are produced by Hay House. To all the professionals and practitioners who helped me in my journey to get off antidepressants – thank-you. I can't even remember the names of all the professionals I've consulted with over the years, but I will list a few here: Dr. Helen Valerio, Dr. Shaw, Dr. Priya Joshi, Dr. Pankaj Seth, Sophie Hawkins, Beth McLellan, and Tara Thomas – many thanks for your advice, resources, and calming energy. My gratitude goes out to all the yogis and yoginis who have supported and inspired me along the way – especially my fellow YTT teachers and graduates from the Lotus Centre. I also have so many friends and family members – aunts, uncles, cousins, grandparents – who have been like rocks to me. There's no way I could mention you all here. You know who you are. Trust me when I say that your emails, words of support, and phone messages did not go unnoticed (even if I never called you back!). Each and every positive word gave me the energy to keep moving forward with this book.

To my mom Lois-Anne – you are the main reason I believe in myself. You provided me with unconditional love throughout my life – even when it looked like others had abandoned me. You sacrificed so much of your own life to make sure I was loved and cared for. It's this unconditional support that helped me know that as long as I put my mind to it, I can do anything. To my stepfather Paul – I've felt your presence the entire time I've been writing this book. I felt the same way when I was writing my Ph.D. thesis. It's like you're right beside me telling me to follow my dreams and keep pushing forward. I will always remember you for your incredible strength, courage, and determination in the face of adversity – and I forgive the rest.

Finally, to my husband David – I dedicated this book to you because it wouldn't exist without you. You held me in my darkest hours of antidepressant withdrawal, and you helped me see the true beauty that exists within me. When I told you I was going to quit my job to write this book, you didn't show one ounce of fear about our finances. You stood by me the entire time, and you have continued to support me in all that I do. You are the love of my life – let's continue to follow our dreams together.

About the Author

B ethany Butzer, Ph.D. is a Mental Health & Wellness
Advisor who specializes in helping her clients reduce
stress, anxiety, and sadness. She provides life coaching,
workshops, and yoga classes that inspire people to improve
their quality of life, reach their full potential, meet their
goals, and get off antidepressant medication.

Dr. Butzer received her Ph.D. in psychology in 2008
from the University of Western Ontario. Her early research
focused on anxiety and depression. After spending several
years studying psychopathology, she changed her focus to
positive psychology, which emphasizes the development
of human strength and potential. Her recent research
has focused on the psychology of romantic relationships
and the effects of yoga on well-being. Dr. Butzer is also
a certified yoga teacher and has received life coaching
training from the Coaches Training Institute (CTI).

Dr. Butzer has published professional papers in several
leading Psychological journals, including *Personality and*

Social Psychology Bulletin and *Personal Relationships*. She has also won numerous national and international awards for her achievements, such as the Martin E. P. Seligman Award for Outstanding Dissertation Research in Positive Psychology.

A unique aspect of Dr. Butzer's approach is that she combines her professional training with her personal experience to provide services that are both empathetic and effective. She has personally overcome the obstacles of a rocky childhood, anxiety, depression, and a dependence on antidepressant medication. She has experienced grief, loss, abuse, abandonment, burnout, and almost everything in between. She has been to doctors, therapists, psychiatrists, and has tried many forms of alternative health. And she has come out on the other side.

Based on her familiarity with both the dark and light sides of life, Dr. Butzer's style is down to earth and approachable, and she has an extensive knowledge of the services that are available to those in need.

Dr. Butzer's mission is to empower people everywhere to lead the *amazing* lives they deserve.

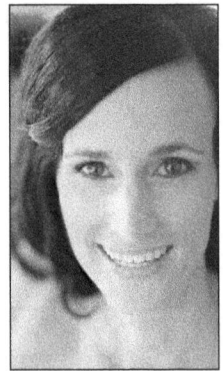

Visit Dr. Butzer's website at
www.bethanybutzer.com.